MULTIAMORY

MULTIAMORY

ESSENTIAL TOOLS
for
MODERN RELATIONSHIPS

DEDEKER WINSTON

JASE LINDGREN

EMILY SOTELO MATLACK

CLEiS
PRESS

Published in the United States by Cleis Press, an imprint of Start Midnight, LLC, 221 River Street, Ninth Floor, Hoboken, New Jersey 07030.

Printed in the United States
Cover design: Britney Walters
Cover illustration: Britney Walters
Text design: Frank Wiedemann

First Edition.
10 9 8 7 6 5 4 3 2 1

Trade paper ISBN: 978-1-62778-320-0
E-book ISBN: 978-1-62778-533-4

TABLE OF CONTENTS

Foreword

I know I'm not the only one who's ever been listening to an episode of *Multiamory* and thought, *Damn, I should really be writing this down.* But never, not once in my many years of being a chronic overachiever and listening to this incredibly useful relationship podcast have I actually pulled out a notebook. I'm usually driving or walking when I'm listening—not sitting at a desk! So instead, I hope the hosts' detailed and savvy advice will stick around in the recesses of my brain for the next time I need it. And while some of it certainly has, unfortunately, apparently not enough that I avoided the hot mess communication situation I depict in my memoir *Open*.

So you can imagine my excitement when I found out that *Multiamory* was coming out with a book that summarized their most important relationship communication advice. Now, finally, their elaborate-yet-simple acronyms would be gathered in one printed place for me to pick up off the shelf as a reference the next time I find myself in conflict with a partner or simply wanting to invest in our relationship's long-term health. *Multiamory:*

Essential Tools for Modern Relationships is a highly curated collection of the most popular communication tools, advice, and lessons from the podcast—and the brilliant hosts behind it.

When I read the book you hold in your hands, I was so thrilled I underlined over half of it (which, admittedly, sort of defeats the purpose of highlighting). What excited me was not just that so much of *Multiamory*'s excellent advice—on boundaries, on listening, on doing the relationship check-in method RADAR, and so much else—was now combined in one convenient print package, but also something perhaps even more meaningful. Here, finally, was a book where nonmonogamous and monogamous relationship advice could truly coexist. Here was a book I would find useful in periods where there are three partners *and* periods when there is only one partner (as of this writing, sadly true, please DM me and try to woo me, seriously, wtf). Here was a book I could also recommend to my monogamous friends, knowing they would feel included and helped while *also* learning a little something about nonmonogamy in the process. A relationship advice book that, for perhaps the first time, nonmonogamous or monogamous, queer or straight, I didn't feel in any way excluded me or anyone I love.

This is a book for anyone who wants to learn how to communicate better, in any aspect of their life. It is for *Multiamory* superfans, and it is for anyone who's never heard of the podcast and doesn't have time to listen to eight years and over 250 episodes of archives.

Over the years, *Multiamory* has gotten more and more inclusive of *all* relationship models, and this book reflects that. They aim to help us communicate and love each other better—no matter how many partners we have, whether we believe in relationship anarchy or prefer hierarchies, swinging, monogamy, or the many myriad options in between. There is an embracing of fluidity and openness to this book—and a refreshing lack of judgment. Unfortunately, when it comes to relationship advice, that is very rare.

Drawing on their years of research on evidence-based relationship advice and feedback, *Multiamory* stirs up all-too-often hetero- and mononormative relationship advice and serves it up in a remixed way that excludes no orientation or relationship model—so long as it's consensual and respectful. This is a book that will not assume you want to get married, choose one gender to be or be with, find "the one," or have kids—nor will it assume that there is something "unevolved" about you if you do want those things. It will not assume your relationship orientation or sexual orientation has to stay fixed throughout your life, or that breaking up is a failure to be avoided at all costs. (In fact, as they refreshingly repeat several times, "It's okay to break up!") It won't even assume you will use this book for romantic relationships (I found the chapter on boundaries particularly useful for communication with my parents, for example).

This book is also a good litmus test. You know that John Waters quote, "If you go home with somebody and they don't have any books, don't fuck 'em"? Well, I would add, "If you're in a relationship with somebody and they refuse to look at this book or try any of its exercises together, don't fuck 'em."

I already trusted my partner would be down to try anything new and useful. Unlike past long-term nonmonogamous relationships, I like to think this one has pretty good communication. It tends to be a low-conflict dynamic, and perhaps for that reason, we both easily agreed that doing a RADAR once a month would be an investment in the relationship's continued health. I'd heard about *Multiamory*'s famous method for relationship check-ins, RADAR, for many years now and thought (also for years) *I should really get around to doing that . . . maybe when I finally take some notes.* But it wasn't until I had this physical book in my hands that I finally put a RADAR check-in on the calendar as a recurring monthly event with my partner.

During our first session, things were expressed and communicated directly that I hadn't even realized had never been made explicit. A safe container to talk about all the hardest and most fun and awkward things had been created easily with this road map. Our sex life, communication about money and the future, and our sense of teamwork—none of which I necessarily had any urgent "problems" with—all improved immediately nonetheless after doing RADAR. And I'm sure that the more we use the tools in this book, the more it can only help reveal the truth and potential of what is already there.

Multiamory's wisdom will be helpful to you in good times and hard times, polyamorous or monogamous, or anything in between. Good communication, mutual respect, love, and compassion never go out of style. And neither will this book.

—Rachel Krantz

Multiamory

From the Latin prefix *multi*, meaning multiple, and the Latin root *amor*, meaning love.

Multiamory represents multiple forms of love—everything from monogamy to nonmonogamy, casual dating to queerplatonic, married couples to those who are single by choice, and everything in between.

| What Is Good Communication?

Love. Intimacy. Companionship. For so many of us, the prospect of finding someone to couple and spend our days with marks the pinnacle of our relationship goals. We are pestered our whole lives by songs, TV shows, and novels about how vital it is to find a mate. Over and over again we watch the familiar boy-meets-girl trope play out on the screen. These shiny stories so often center around the perils of wooing a prospective partner, overcoming obstacles, and finally "getting the girl." Triumphantly, the couple eventually comes together, the credits roll, and everyone lives happily ever after in bliss and harmony. Cheerful moviegoers leave the theater without ever asking the question "What now? What happens next?"

What happens next isn't always as lighthearted and joyous as those movies would lead us to believe. It's commonplace for misunderstandings, baggage from old loves, and miscommunication to plague almost every relationship at one time or another. If left unchecked, these issues can lead to insecurity, resentment, anxiety, and shame. The relationship may ultimately fizzle out or ignite into a big blowup and end, leaving us wondering, "Where did it all go wrong?"

We, your authors, Jase, Dedeker, and Emily, have been there, too. It wasn't long ago that the three of us were navigating the murky waters of bad relationships, crappy first dates, and unmet expectations. Conflict and explosive emotions were par for the course. Maybe you'll recognize some of your own relationship mishaps in our stories.

EMILY SAYS

It was March 2010. I had just returned to my final quarter of college in Cincinnati after a spring break trip home with my boyfriend. We had only been dating for three months, but I was head over heels in love with the guy. We had so much fun, the sex was great, and he was absolutely adorable. I had a blast showing him off to all my friends and family the previous week when we were together in Tucson. I was leaving my undergraduate program in less than a month, while he was due to stay in Cincinnati getting his master's for another year or two. I pushed the upcoming prospect of a long-distance relationship out of my mind for the time being. We were great together, enjoying each other's company, and, besides—he was perfect! We would make it work. What could possibly go wrong?

The week after we got back, he dumped me. He said he had been contemplating doing it before our trip but decided against it because I was *obviously* so excited to have him meet my friends and family. He agreed the sex was awesome, but I was leaving soon, and we were just "having fun." And, most egregiously, it was clear to him that I was way more into him than he was into me. It wasn't cool or sexy to him, so it was time for the relationship to end.

Needless to say, I was shocked and devastated. I was so infatuated with him that it was impossible for me to see the writing on the wall. I should have raised an eyebrow at all the noncommittal answers to my friends' questions when they asked what his favorite thing was about me or how we were going to stay together once I moved away after college. I should have realized we didn't have that much in common and that most of our quality time together was spent between the sheets. But mostly I should have recognized that we never had an honest discussion about how we really felt about one another, what we each wanted out of the relationship, and what our plans were for the future.

Each of us had an internal story about the nature of the relationship that was completely opposite! He was looking for a fun, short-term fling, and I was looking for someone to fill the massive, companion-sized hole in my heart. Neither of us was wrong for what we wanted, but both of us failed to communicate our true feelings and intentions. This was certainly not the first time something like this had happened to me, and the pattern of burying my head in the sand and failing to communicate my wants and needs to my partners would continue for many years to come.

JASE SAYS

In my twenties, after being together for almost two years, my girlfriend and I decided to get engaged. We got along incredibly well, and it was the lowest-conflict relationship I'd had up to that point. She felt the same way, so we decided to buy each other rings and planned on a long engagement before getting married. I felt like I had it all figured out: I had cracked the code of relationships and was finally getting my happily ever after. This relationship was a source of pride at how I'd managed to find someone who really got me, who was fun and social, and who encouraged me to succeed. We traveled together for six months and then moved to Seattle to start figuring out our careers and lives.

Over the following year, things were challenging as we both tried to find work. She tried several different jobs, which didn't work out for one reason or another, and I ended up going to beauty school to become a hairstylist. We both did our best to support and encourage each other despite any challenges that arose. During those explorations, we each learned new skills, found new interests, and made new friends, but we also began to drift apart from one another. It's easy to realize after the fact, but at the time I thought everything was fine. We were having a lot less sex, and we had more disagreements while living in a one-bedroom apartment together, but that seemed normal. It was just part of the process of settling down and establishing a life.

Our communication was good when it came to talking about other people, politics, or more philosophical topics, but we struggled to effectively share our own inner journeys as we explored our careers and made friends in a new city.

Growth is an essential part of life, no matter your age, but we were failing to share that growth with each other.

After a year and a half of being engaged, we broke up with "I love you, but I'm not in love with you anymore," and she moved back to the Midwest. I was heartbroken that I'd lost the relationship, but it was also a huge hit to my pride. I had been so sure that I had figured it out and had won the relationship game. I was so quick to brag to others about my success that when it all fell apart, I was ashamed and embarrassed on top of all the hurt and sadness. I had fallen into the trap of identifying with my relationship as a status symbol—a marker of success for a well-adjusted member of society. The breakup took me years to recover from.

DEDEKER SAYS

I literally couldn't speak. I was shivering on the front lawn of my high school, staring daggers at my friend Miguel (Friend? Boyfriend? Even that hadn't been clearly communicated between us). I don't even remember the content of our falling-out that day, but I remember that I was upset, angry, sad, and feeling a billion other emotions that I needed him to hear, but my teeth were glued together. I remember his perplexed face as he asked question after question, trying to get something out of me, but I was a statue. It wasn't that I wanted to give him the silent treatment. This wasn't a punishment or a manipulation. It was just the only way that I knew how to be in the face of turbulent emotions. Somewhere between my brain and my mouth, there was blaring static, a signal too fuzzy for the muscles of my lips and tongue to even parse in the first place. Even if I could open my mouth, all that would come out would be either incoherent gibberish, a primal wail, or, worst of all—a stumbling yet honest account of what I was feeling and what I wanted. For any of the above to escape would usher in a fate worse than death, so my jaw remained wired shut.

Some version of this interaction plagued every subsequent adult relationship I had. Over time I learned to fine-tune it. It turns out that emotional freeze-outs and verbal shutdowns work nicely for the moments where you do want to punish or manipulate someone. This communication approach set me up for a real bind: I had to avoid upset feelings and relationship conflict at all costs. The only way to accomplish this was to find a partner who could provide what I wanted and who could make me feel safe and loved. I couldn't reliably express what I wanted or ask for what would make me feel safe and loved, so I had to hope against hope that maybe in my next relationship I'd finally find someone who already knew all this information without me having to tell them.

This slowly became my definition of compatibility, not based on personalities, communication styles, or alignment of life goals and values, but on something more elusive and impossibly magical. Magic is an essential line item on the bill of goods we're all sold, assured that these are the only ingredients needed for the love of a lifetime. I recall plenty of magical mind reading and grand romantic gestures in the Disney films and rom-coms of my youth. What's harder to recall is any scene where the princess vulnerably asks the prince if they can set up a weekly date night.

We have each had our fair share of breakups, breakdowns, and breakthroughs in our personal relationship journeys. At some point each of us had a similar thought, one that you may have had yourself: there has to be a better way. There has to be something out there that could solve these problems, or at least help to avoid having so many of them. There had to be some tip or trick that would help break bad habits and move us toward healthier and happier partnerships, rather than doing the same thing over and over again in the hope that it would someday get better.

The *Multiamory* Podcast: Origin Story

In the midst of these negative relationship routines and habitual toxicity, the three of us yearned for something different. Jase and Emily met not long after she moved to Los Angeles and spent two and a half years in a traditional, monogamous relationship. After a brief separation, they realized they were interested in exploring what other people had to offer emotionally and sexually yet wanted to maintain the intimate companionship that they still had with each other. It was the decision to break away from traditional monogamy and a foray into polyamory that eventually led Jase and Emily to meet Dedeker, who was already in the midst of her own polyamorous journey with another partner. We all stumbled through many exciting and scary firsts: meeting metamours (our partners' other partners), experimenting with triad and quad relationships, and many other different, subversive, and novel ways of relating.

It was during this time, back in 2014, that the *Multiamory* podcast was born. We knew there were many people besides those in our social sphere who were also practicing nonmonogamy, but we didn't know just how prevalent it had become. Polls suggest at least one in five Americans has practiced some form of consensual nonmonogamy in their lifetime. Yet, there were still few resources available at the time on how to conduct healthy polyamorous relationships. Additionally, many traditional relationship advice shows were advocating incredibly toxic and unhealthy practices (and sadly many still do today). Most of the relationship advice we found was based solely on traditional, mainstream views of how relationships should look and geared primarily toward people seeking a monogamous, long-term commitment. We craved information that dared to explore new ways of thinking about relationships with an emphasis on psychology, neuroscience, and research. Planning, writing, and recording weekly episodes of the podcast led us to research from other leaders in the relationship field, and we began crafting unique tools to better our own relationships as well as those of our budding listenership.

As time went on, we began to notice how many of the things we were discussing in the polyamorous space echoed many of our experiences when we were monogamous. We heard from listeners in traditional relationships that they were also finding value from hearing about polyamorous approaches to crafting relationships. Our deeply nonmonogamous podcast started to shift to include all forms of love, from consciously chosen monogamy to ethical polyamory, queerplatonic friendships, chosen family, relationship anarchy, and more. (If you aren't familiar with some of these terms, don't worry. The point is, there are a lot of different ways to do relationships!) Our community grew, and we were able to gain wisdom and feedback from others whose experiences were different from our own. We learn right along with our listeners every day, and we have continued to adjust and fine-tune the ways in which we approach and experience communication in our own relationships.

The landscape of our own bonds with one another has changed over the course of creating the podcast. Emily and Jase are no longer in a romantic relationship, yet Jase and Dedeker remain in a polyamorous relationship together. Emily, on the other hand, has been happily monogamous with her partner, Josh, for many years. Our collective years of experience with many different types of relationships (and making all kinds of huge mistakes along the way) have been instrumental in the ongoing health of our individual connections, as well as the ongoing partnership between the three of us. However you choose to identify your romantic relationships, the tools outlined here can enact meaningful and positive changes.

There is no shortage of relationship advice bombarding us in the form of podcasts, books, blogs, articles, counselors, and weeklong retreats. Some of it is fabulous, and some is surprisingly unhealthy. When something piques our interest, we've taken a closer look into that advice to see if it will resonate well with our audience. Through trial and error, we've found that so much of the wisdom out there is often difficult to integrate into one's life in a practical way, or it's simply geared toward only one specific type of relationship. Our goal has been to tailor communication tools so that they are effective no matter what type of relationship you are in, simple enough to understand, and easy to remember and apply in your daily life. If we can make it into an acronym somehow, even better!

Our hope for readers of this book is the same hope we hold for everyone who listens to the podcast. Whether you are monogamous, polyamorous, swinging, casually dating, or if you just want to do relationships differently, we hope you can use these tools and lessons to have better relationships with others and with yourself. We see you, and we're here for you. Now, let's dive into some key concepts that will be important for the journey ahead!

Why should we strive for good communication?

Good communication is essential for healthy relationships. Without it, we face the constant struggle of our own internal stories about why our partner thinks and behaves the way they do, and we are subject to our partner's internal stories as well. It can become extraordinarily irritating to play guessing games about why a partner said something a certain way, why they seem upset, or what it is that they want out of their life in the next five years. Yet most media outlets tell us that an ideal union occurs when you and your partner are so well matched that you intuitively know exactly what each other is thinking. In reality, learning to read your partner's mind is an impossible goal, resulting in hurt, frustration, and failure, and we argue that it should be stricken from the world's lists of relationship goals!

Instead, we should be seeking more effective ways to listen to our partners, asking sincere questions about their state of being, and cultivating compassion for the things that bring about painful emotions. Our partners evolve and change throughout the course of a relationship, just like we do. Their thoughts and feelings about things that were important to them when you began your relationship may develop and shift over time. We are all fluid and dynamic creatures and can't expect our own needs or the needs of our partners to stay static throughout the trajectory of the relationship. The ability to communicate those fluctuating needs, thoughts, desires, and feelings is key.

But don't just take our word for it! In 2021, researchers Terri Conley and Jennifer Piemonte, from the University of Michigan, published a paper combining the results of five studies of couples in different types of nonmonogamous relationships. When analyzing the collected results, they found that good communication skills were one of the most significant factors in predicting relationship satisfaction. As they wrote in the paper, "those who use more effective communication strategies and know their partners' partners better have better outcomes." Our communication patterns can clearly show the health of our relationships, too. Dr. John Gottman and the Gottman Institute can make wildly accurate predictions of whether or not a couple will break up by simply observing the couple discuss a conflict for fifteen minutes. While many other things can drastically affect relationship satisfaction, including money problems, environmental stress, positive or negative interaction, and individual personality traits, communication is one of the most vital areas that can make or break a relationship.

What is a relationship?

In order to talk about improving relationships, it is worth taking a moment to clarify what we mean by "relationship." For most people, the word *relationship* brings to mind dating, romance, and sex, yet we have relationships with every single person we come into contact with (some more brief than others). You have a relationship with your mail carrier, with your neighbor, with your family members, and with your coworkers. You even have a relationship with us by reading this book or listening to our podcast! Clearly, these connections are not all the same. Some may be much closer than others, some may involve physical touch, some may be more intentional, and others may be circumstantial.

The tools we present in this book are meant to improve every relationship, which means they don't have to be limited to just romantic or sexual relationships. In the following chapters, we often use romantic couples as examples, and we usually refer to the people involved as partners, but these tools can be applied to any intentional relationship. You may not sit down for a relationship check-in conversation with your mail carrier, but you certainly could with your sister or a close friend. Communication is the lifeblood of any close partnership, whether that involves physical intimacy, romance, or none of the above. At the end of the day, we get to choose which relationships we want to enhance and cultivate, and we get to work together with others to determine how we want to foster the relationship, regardless of their external category. We like how philosopher and author Carrie Jenkins puts it: "What I call 'eudaemonic' (good-spirited) love can be thought of as a creative project—the collaborative telling of a new story. It is not about the passive acceptance of existing scripts."

As you read the tools in this book, be sure to spend some time thinking about the various relationships in your life to evaluate which tools may be a good fit.

What is relationship success?

This may seem like a simple question, but it is actually one of the core challenges in relationship research and education. Traditionally, when it came to measuring the success of a romantic relationship, the only metric used was time—the longer the relationship, the more successful it is. We tend to think that if a relationship lasts a long time, it's a success, and if it only lasts a short time, then it is a failure. Based on this very narrow definition of success, we can end up glorifying a fifty-year relationship full of abuse, lying, manipulation, and general misery over a six-month relationship based on honesty, compassion, and joy. Don't get us wrong— having a long-lasting, caring, happy relationship is fantastic, but when we get too focused on duration, we can lose sight of what truly makes relationships healthy.

Our culture encourages us to become goal oriented in our intimate relationships. We may focus on hitting specific milestones or markers of commitment, rather than questioning whether the relationship itself is a positive influence in our own life as well as our partner's. Do you know someone who perceives their relationship this way and is hyperfocused on their goals of getting to the next step, whether moving in together, getting married, or having a baby? They may get short-lived fulfillment from pursuing their goals, only to eventually have a rude awakening once they achieve them. Sadly, their enthusiasm for the relationship may dissolve once they don't have another goal to pursue.

Author Amy Gahran calls this phenomenon "the relationship escalator" and argues, "The Relationship Escalator is one of many *social scripts*—customs for how people are 'supposed' to behave, and how we 'should' think or feel in certain contexts, situations or interactions. These customs benefit many people, but not always, and not everyone." She also spoke on how the one-size-fits-all escalator mentality that many counselors, books, and podcasts adhere to can ultimately harm those who aren't in pursuit of that type of relationship: "Assuming that the traditional Relationship Escalator is the only type of important intimate relationship that people should have or want reinforces the strong social privilege available only to couples on the Escalator."

While we agree that it's important to have personal and shared goals, we strive to help listeners, clients, and ourselves refocus relationship pursuits by bringing a spirit of inquiry. "Eight billion people cannot fit under one way of living," says Michelle Hy, nonmonogamy advocate and creator of the Polyamorous While Asian Instagram account. "While it can feel daunting, it's helpful to remember that because each of us has decades of mono- and amatonormative programming to sift through; relearning will not happen overnight. Everyone's timeline is different, and the least we can do is to remain actively curious. Why are you in the relationships you're in? If no one cared or judged you, what would your relationships (with others and with yourself) look like? Are these structures serving you, or are you serving the idea of these structures?"

> ## WHAT THE HECK DOES "AMATONORMATIVE" MEAN?
>
> If you've never heard this term before, don't worry! The term *amatonormativity* was coined by Dr. Elizabeth Brake to describe the societal pressure to pursue a romantic, sexual, long-term monogamous relationship, especially marriage, and the assumption that everyone wants the same thing. In her writings, she uses the term to point out how this assumption minimizes and invalidates people who don't fit that one mold, such as asexual, aromantic, or nonmonogamous people, and causes us to treat single people as incomplete and somehow lacking.
>
> A similar term, *mononormative*, is used for the assumption that monogamous relationships are the only valid or worthwhile relationships and that anyone who isn't in one should be seeking to enter one.

What is a healthy relationship?

When we talk about healthy relationships, what do we mean? Loveisrespect.org, a national resource to prevent abuse and intimate partner violence, uses the acronym REST to describe healthy relationships. REST stands for Respect, Equality, Safety, and Trust. We believe these four words should be the baseline for what a healthy relationship looks like. In other words, both partners consistently respecting each other, working to create an equal and fair partnership, feeling safe with their partner, and being trustworthy are not relationship goals, but the *bare minimum* we should expect from our relationships. Sadly, there are many relationships out there that do not meet this standard. If you're in a relationship where one or all of these pillars are missing, we encourage and advocate for you to examine your relationship and see if it is causing more harm than good. As we say all the time on the show, it's okay to break up.

On the other hand, if your relationship has hit a snag that you can't seem to untangle, if you and your partner feel apathy creeping in, or if you experience a myriad of little fights and want to break an unhealthy pattern, the tools in this book will help steer you back in the right direction. Our goal is to give you lasting advice on how to alter the way in which you connect with your partners on a fundamental level, and infuse more support, kindness, affection, and love—basically all the good stuff that make relationships a joy. Ultimately, healthy communication can turn a decent relationship into an amazing one and can help us to respectfully end or change our unhealthy relationships so we can focus more on ones that truly lift us up.

What to expect in this book

This book has taken on many different iterations in the writing process. Initially it was going to be a companion to the entire *Multiamory* episode catalog (literally impossible to do when you're producing new episodes every week). Then it was going to be a manual solely focused on RADAR, our template for creating monthly relationship check-ins with partners (which ended up as Chapter 7). Where we've arrived is a book that's part companion and part tool kit. We've tried to design this book to be as approachable as possible, whether you've listened to every single *Multiamory* episode, only a handful, or none at all. And just like our podcast, you may find it best to read straight from beginning to end, or you may find it more useful to check the Table of Contents and jump around to the tools that will be the most effective for your current situation. Let's look at what you can expect as you make your way through this book.

ROAD MAP TO THE TOOLS

Here's a sneak preview of each tool you'll encounter:

- CHAPTER 2: The Triforce of Communication—Here's where you'll learn how to metacommunicate and get what you actually need out of conversations through three specific, easy-to-use communication approaches.

- CHAPTER 3: Spewers and Chewers—This chapter lays out the fine points of internal and external processing and will help you determine your personal processing style, including strategies to use if your partner's style is similar to or different from your own.

- CHAPTER 4: Microscripts—In this chapter you'll learn how to create short, predetermined interactions between you and your partner to interrupt old patterns, defuse tension, create new habits, and act as a shortcut to healthier communication.

- CHAPTER 5: Boundaries—We dispel common misconceptions about what boundaries are and when they should be used and provide an exercise for determining your own true boundaries. You'll also learn to use our SELF tool to create actionable, unilateral ways to enforce your boundaries with others and, even more importantly, with yourself.

- CHAPTER 6: Repair SHOP—You will learn a process for coming back together after conflict so that a disagreement or argument can actually encourage growth rather than destruction and resentment.

- CHAPTER 7: RADAR—This chapter will cover RADAR, a check-in formula for regularly maintaining the health of your relationships. This framework has been life changing for many of us and will help you and your partner collaborate on creating your ideal relationship.

- EXTRA TOOLS—This is a collection of short summaries of additional tools created by others that have been instrumental to our own communication practices, as well as a few more of our own tools and concepts.

- REFERENCES—Any books, studies, or other resources we mention throughout this book can be found in the references section. We also provide more details about all our special guests so you can look them up and support their work.

PERSONAL STORIES

We've done our best to include stories that involve real-life applications for each tool. In addition to our personal experiences, we also share narratives based on real-world experiences told to us by our listeners. Most stories use pseudonyms and may have details changed or have multiple stories blended together in order to preserve privacy.

MULTIPLE RELATIONSHIP STYLES, MULTIPLE VIEWPOINTS

Over the years, our scope has broadened as we strive to create relationship resources that are as inclusive as possible. We aim to acknowledge and incorporate some of the additional complexities of nonmonogamy alongside concerns felt in monogamous relationships. Throughout this book, you'll find examples and anecdotes from a mix of different relationship viewpoints, including polyamory, various different forms of nonmonogamy, as well as traditional monogamy. When we use the word *partner*, that may refer to a spouse, lover, best friend, an exclusive romantic connection, or just one of many people in a polycule.

Being exposed to different relationship practices may bring up challenging feelings. For you hard-core polyamorous folks, it may mean setting aside judgment toward monogamous relationships and trying to generate some empathy. For monogamous folks, this may mean examining any feelings of alarm, discomfort, or intrigue that come up when presented with nonmainstream ways of relating. For heterosexual and cisgender readers, that might mean uncomfortable exposure to challenges that you may not have faced in your own life. We want to create a world that has room for many different relationship formats with many different types of people, and we hope that you can help us in that pursuit. As Amy Gahran, author of *Stepping Off the Relationship Escalator*, says, "Important personal intimate relationships have never, ever been one size fits all. Recognizing and embracing this reality of diversity simply makes you . . . realistic." We encourage you to give yourself the chance to learn from relationships and people whose lives and loves may look very different from your own.

With that in mind, this is not a book about polyamory, and we will not cover subjects like how to open up your relationship for the first time, navigating jealousy, or where to find potential partners. There are many wonderful books out there on the subject, including Dedeker's first book, *The Smart Girl's Guide to Polyamory*. The tools and tips in this book apply to any kind of relationship and have been thoroughly tested by us and our listeners in both monogamous and nonmonogamous partnerships.

SPECIAL GUESTS

The work of some of our favorite people in the relationship-betterment field is discussed often on our podcast and will be referenced throughout this book. While we've created some of our own tools from scratch or changed an existing tool into something more practical and comprehensive for our audience, there are also many tools from others that we discuss and utilize on a regular basis. In addition to our own experiences and the knowledge we've gained from our clients and listeners over the years, our guests each add their own perspectives, and we hope you enjoy getting to learn from their insights. You will find quotes throughout this book from many other educators, writers, researchers, and therapists who regularly use our tools and others who have inspired us.

TAKEAWAYS AND HOMEWORK

There is a lot of great information in this book and floating around in the relationship advice space, but it goes to waste if we don't find specific ways to incorporate that knowledge into our individual lives. At the end of each chapter, you'll find a list of key concepts to remember as well as quick reference guides when applicable. These can act as a cheat sheet for when these tools get put to the test in real life. We've also included homework at the end of each chapter in the form of journal prompts or exercises to further drive home each concept and provide a pathway for applying them to your relationships.

BONUS: A GRAB BAG OF TOOLS!

There's a fun bonus in the last chapter: a big ol' grab bag of tools, tips, guidance, and other wisdom that we've found particularly useful. Some of it comes from us, but most of it comes from other great thinkers and educators that have inspired us over the years. If we mention a tool or concept that you're unfamiliar with, it's likely there is a more thorough explanation in the Extra Tools chapter. We'll include information in each section as to where you can find more in-depth details regarding each tool.

Before We Begin

We cannot overstate the power of incorporating intentional check-ins, an understanding of your processing style, and clear meta-communication into your relationships. But we also don't want to set up the expectation that these tools are cure-alls. Sadly, this is not a book of magic spells (we'll start working on a grimoire of our own once we've launched our next podcast, *Multisorcery*). These are some important truths to bear in mind as you begin applying these tools to your relationships.

EVEN THE BEST COMMUNICATION TOOL IN THE WORLD CAN'T FORCE SOMEONE TO COMMUNICATE IF THEY DON'T WANT TO.

We don't have any secret manipulative devices to get your partners to open up and share their vulnerabilities. We can't promise that if you just use this *one weird trick* your partner will always be forthright and honest. There's no special text-message template to guarantee your new crush will finally text you back. However, the content of this book will help you *create the conditions* that make it easier to open up and share the scary, tender stuff, easier to be honest even when it's awkward, and easier to let go when someone isn't communicating the way you'd prefer them to.

Someone who "refuses to communicate" is probably not just being stubborn for the sake of stubbornness. An aversion or inability to communicate can often be an indicator that the person doesn't know how to talk about a particular topic. They may have never had this kind of conversation modeled for them. This particular subject may have been taboo where they grew up. They might be too scared or overwhelmed by the topic. They may feel too much hurt and trauma regarding the topic, so much so that they don't think they can open their mouth without falling apart. They may think the topic will not be received in a gentle or compassionate way. There are a million reasons why communication is difficult in general, and our own individual experiences, preferences, and hang-ups complicate it even further. If there is someone in your life who refuses to communicate, get curious, and to the best of your ability, get compassionate. At the end of the day, though, you can't do someone else's personal growth for them.

EVEN THE BEST COMMUNICATION TOOL IN THE WORLD CAN BE MISUSED AND ABUSED.

We've heard countless stories of people giving up after trying all kinds of techniques: nonviolent communication, countless forms of couples' counseling, active listening, and even some of our own tools. Usually, the negative experience is tied to a partner's bad behavior, using an allegedly "healthy" communication technique to perpetuate unhealthy patterns of control.

Unfortunately, this is all too easy to do. Even with good intentions, any tool can be misunderstood or misapplied, leading to confusion or hurt feelings. At worst, a particular communication framework can be used intentionally to justify making unfair demands, belittling a partner, or gaslighting. There is even precedent that suggests otherwise healthy communication tools or couples' therapy may make an already abusive relationship even worse.

How can we prevent this? To start, focus on connecting to your deeper purpose for wanting to communicate at all. Chances are high that you're craving safety, security, closeness, understanding, compassion, or collaboration—all good things that are fundamental to healthy relationships. Let that be your guiding light, and if the way a tool is being used is getting in the way of that, either customize or set it aside for now. You might also consider consulting individually with a trusted professional such as a counselor or coach to help determine if you may be in an unhealthy dynamic.

EVEN THE BEST COMMUNICATION TOOL IN THE WORLD CAN FAIL TO "FIX" INCOMPATIBILITIES OR RESCUE A DYSFUNCTIONAL RELATIONSHIP.

The sad reality is that many people don't start thinking about communicating intentionally until there is already a backlog of problems and a track record of bad habits. That doesn't mean that it's too late to make a change, but the path ahead may require a lot of hard work. That being said, it's unlikely there is a single tool, book, therapist, or approach that can miraculously erase set-in patterns overnight, and be wary of anyone that makes such claims. Again, we want to encourage you to enlist the help of a trusted friend, family member, or therapist to help explore the possibility that your relationship may not be serving you anymore. Sometimes it's best to end the relationship and appreciate it for all the lessons it has taught you while moving forward in search of something healthier and less fraught with conflict and pain. If you are starting from a place of knowing that your relationship is healthy enough to be worth improving, then congratulations! You are already much more likely to build an amazing, life-affirming relationship.

WE LOVE RESEARCH! BUT RESEARCH HAS ITS LIMITS.
On the show and in this book, we strive to include as much
evidence-based advice and research findings as we can. While not
all relationship advice has to be empirically supported by hard
science in order to be valid, looking at research can help answer
some important questions. Is this common relationship advice
actually bullshit? Or is there a grain of truth to it? Are there
factors influencing my relationships, communication, or mental
health that I'm not even aware of? In a landscape now inundated
with competing opinions about what truly makes relationships
work, studies, surveys, and various forms of analyses can help to
draw a distinction between the helpful and the unhelpful. We try
to incorporate the best of both worlds: tried-and-true relationship
wisdom combined with evidence-based approaches.

However, even research is limited. Historically, researchers
have recruited study participants from a homogenous population
of undergrad students, often wholly excluding people of color;
women; people with disabilities; nonbinary, trans, and queer
folks; people in consensually nonmonogamous relationships;
happily single people; willingly unmarried people, and the list
goes on and on. We are seeing this start to shift in recent years,
but remember that some research findings may not be completely
applicable to everyone.

In addition, directions of correlation and causation in research
can often be sensationalized and misconstrued, usually by the
media. This pops up in relationship research all the time. A particular study may find that cooking and eating dinner together with
a partner on a regular basis is correlated with a higher average
household income. What usually happens next is that a media
outlet will pounce on the study and publish a headline to the tune
of MAKE DINNER FOR YOUR GIRLFRIEND IF YOU WANT TO BE
RICH!!!

The problem is this fictional study hasn't established that cooking dinner together *causes* the household income to rise. It only establishes that these two things are *associated* with each other. Further research is needed to clarify what's actually going on here—do people who eat dinner together have a more calm, stable home life, and that's what contributes to better job performance and thus higher income? Or do these people already have a higher income, which enables them to have the extra resources necessary to buy good ingredients, in addition to having the free time to dedicate to cooking? We encourage you to be on the lookout for correlation-causation mix-ups in any research that you encounter in articles, blogs, clickbait news stories, or even daily conversation!

Good research is uncovering new findings every day, as well as recognizing its own limitations. In time, some of the research we cite in this book may be contradicted or replaced by newer studies. Beware of any claims that something is "scientifically proven"—there is no such thing, and everything is subject to revision and reanalysis. This is fundamental to the scientific process, and that's a good thing!

REMEMBER TO CUSTOMIZE . . .

There is no one-size-fits-all communication tool, which is why we encourage everyone to call on their inner creative forces and customize a tool to fit the person you are today and the relationship you are in today. You know your strengths and weaknesses, and you probably know your partner's strengths and weaknesses as well. Some tools in this book may feel clunky and inorganic until you find ways to make them your own. Most of this book is written with intimate partnerships in mind, but we encourage you to find ways to use these tools with family, friends, coworkers, or in any relationship where you're seeking better communication. Ultimately, any tool you use should be serving the real purpose and longing underneath it. Like we said above, getting clear on your purpose will give you clues about the best ways to customize any particular tool.

. . . DON'T WEAPONIZE!

Please don't misuse these tools. We created them with a foundation of kindness and compassion, serving the ultimate purpose of making it easier to listen, understand, and connect deeply with the people you love. However, as we stated before, many communication tools can also be manipulated and twisted to cause harm rather than help. If you find this starting to happen, or a particular tool isn't working for you, engage your creativity to see if you can customize it to a better fit. If it's still not working, scrap it altogether. We won't be offended. There are thousands of techniques, approaches, tips, and tricks for improving communication and handling relationship friction. We would rather you explore and find what works for you and the relationship you are in today rather than force one of our tools to work when it clearly is not.

Go forth!

We are so excited to share this book and our customizable tools with you now. While we truly appreciate those of you who are fans of our work, you certainly don't need to be one of our listeners to get something out of this book. Our hope is that regardless of your background and relationship configuration, you will find these tools to be a fantastic jumping-off point for you and your partners in times of struggle, apathy, and even moments of joy. We strive to go beyond the conventional tips, tricks, and quick fixes of other relationship advice models and instead dig deeper into where your values, ethics, and beliefs lie to help you turn to them for guidance when situations get challenging. If at first you don't succeed, try not to get discouraged! We've personally used these tools hundreds and hundreds of times, and while we still have moments of communication mishaps, they have become less frequent the more we have practiced communicating intentionally. There will always be unexpected moments when it comes to engaging in intimate relationships, but often those challenges can be a catalyst for each of you to break through into new levels of understanding and affection. So, if you are ready, strap in, hold on, and get ready to elevate your relationships in ways you never thought possible!

Homework

We're hitting the ground running with a journal exercise before we even get to the good stuff. Before embarking on this journey, it's important to connect to your *why*. Take a moment to reflect on why you picked up this book (if the reason is "because *Multiamory* is the best," that's okay by us). But beyond being our biggest fan, what's drawing you to the tools in this book? Is there a specific tool that catches your attention? Do you want your partner to read this book or to try out a particular tool? As you read, keep asking questions and drilling down to the foundation of what you are *really* longing for. Understanding your purpose and desires will be the key to understanding the most effective ways to use these tools and how to talk to your partner about using these tools. Here are a few examples to get the juices flowing:

I'm longing for . . .

- a feeling of closeness and safety in my relationships
- a chance to be truly listened to and understood
- my relationship conflicts to feel shorter, easier, and lighter

- the opportunity to know and understand what my partner is thinking and feeling
- ways to honestly express my feelings and desires
- the ability to say no without feeling guilt and shame

With these motivations fresh in your mind, let's continue on to learn about the tools themselves!

CHAPTER 2

The Triforce of Communication:
Go Meta in Your Conversations

Taylor and Sebastian had a solid relationship, but Sebastian's new job was starting to take a toll on them both. Sebastian often needed to work overtime late into the night, sometimes even through the weekend. Taylor was proud of Sebastian for finally getting this new position, and he did his best to be supportive and understanding, even when they had to put their own date night plans on hold.

But there was one night that Taylor finally hit his limit. After several consecutive days of Sebastian needing to postpone or cancel their plans to meet up, Taylor was feeling lonely and frustrated. It was getting harder and harder to listen with compassion whenever Sebastian unpacked his day with him over the phone. He knew he wanted to talk about his frustrations, and he was hoping to get some acknowledgment and empathy from Seb in return.

After Sebastian got home that night, Taylor came over for a late dinner. He was eager to discuss his feelings with Sebastian. Taylor sat down at the dinner table, took a breath, and began,

"Listen, there's something that's been on my mind for a while. I'm happy for you getting this new job, but this past week not being able to see you as much has been incredibly hard for me . . ."

Taylor continued, but Sebastian was stone-faced. He couldn't believe what he was hearing. They had already talked at length about what this job would mean for Sebastian's life, how it would help him finally get out of debt, and they had even strategized on how to make the transition smoother. Seb gritted his teeth until Taylor had finished speaking his piece.

"I've already been clear that I'm not putting in overtime for the rest of this week," he said tersely. "And I've been doing my best to text you during the day and stay in touch. We both acknowledged this would be a tough transition. What else do you want from me?"

Taylor was taken aback. This was not the response he was expecting.

"I . . . I don't know," he said. "I don't think you need to do anything; I'm just saying that it feels lonely sometimes."

"I could try calling more often on my lunch break," he offered, exasperated. "But I can't take a huge chunk out of my workday. I have a hard enough time doing everything I need to do as it is."

"No, that's not what I'm asking for!" Taylor insisted. "I want you to be able to focus on your work. I'm not asking you to change that. But all this overtime has an impact on me, too, and I don't feel like you see that."

"Of course I see that, but there really isn't anything else I can *do* about it!"

The Purposes of Communication

All communication has a purpose. Sometimes the purpose of one's communication is abundantly clear:

"I'm telling you this because I want to come clean."

"I have to take my mom to the doctor today. Do you mind picking up the kids for me?"

"I am sorry for how short I've been toward you in our recent conversations. I've been under a lot of stress at work."

"Multiamory's book is the best thing since sliced bread, and I'm going to tell everyone about it!"

But other times, the purpose of communication can be murkier. In Taylor and Sebastian's story, neither one of them had a clear grasp on what the actual purpose of the conversation was. Taylor may not have known exactly what he was seeking from Sebastian, but he knew that it was *not* what Seb was giving him. Sebastian had an idea of what *he* thought Taylor wanted but felt frustrated and powerless to help him.

Not only were these two unclear about each other's intentions, they were actively communicating at cross-purposes based on assumptions they had made about those intentions. In Sebastian and Taylor's case, it led to needless exasperation, defensiveness, and hurt. At the end of the conversation, neither of them came away having gotten what they wanted.

This is not a newly discovered problem. We've all heard some variation of the Taylor and Sebastian story, especially if you've ever read any other relationship advice book. However, this tale is usually told using conventional stereotypes about gender that started getting moldy decades ago:

LIGHTS COME UP ON A SUBURBAN LIVING ROOM.

The woman comes home and opens up to her male partner about a stressful situation at work. The man, using his hyperrational man brain™, unloads a laundry list of pragmatic sugges- tions for how the woman can fix the situa- tion. The woman succumbs to her emotional lady nature and wells up in frustrated tears because the man isn't listening. The man can't stand feeling relationally impotent and harrumphs his way back to organizing saw blades in the garage.

END SCENE.

While this is usually how the story is presented, there is no real connection between the purpose of communication and someone's gender. It would be incredibly limiting if there were! Rather, all of us have different purposes for our communication at different times based on what we are trying to accomplish or what we need from the other person. Sadly, when that communication doesn't line up with our partner's, it can end up doing the opposite of what we wanted. It's a tale as old as time, repeated regardless of the gender, sexual orientation, or relationship style of the players. Without understanding the purpose behind our own communica- tion, armed only with assumptions about our partner's purposes, we all too often set ourselves up for communication failure.

The Cost of Cross-Purpose Communication

Communicating at cross-purposes brings up a host of problems.

Below are a few examples of how this can show up in your relationship:

DEFENSIVENESS

If your partner gets upset when you offer sympathy at a time when they really wanted advice, it's natural to want to cry, "But I was just trying to help! Why are you mad at me for trying to support you?"

People in healthy relationships are rarely *intending* for communication to go awry. When your partner comes to you hoping you'll listen to their problems, it's unlikely that you're just waiting for a chance to disappoint them. Unfortunately, good intentions don't cancel out the negative impact of communication mishaps. Good intentions can, however, make us all too ready to get defensive when the conversation falls apart.

POWERLESSNESS AND CONFUSION

"I have no idea how to help!"

If you are someone who thrives on problem-solving, there is no worse feeling than powerlessness. You may find yourself throwing out suggestions and advice, only to have each one shot down by an increasingly irritated partner. Even worse, your partner may accept your advice, but their negative feelings about the situation may not go away. Author and therapist Kathy Labriola, who specializes in working with polyamorous and kinky folks, has seen this come up many times. "One partner is experiencing some kind of distress over their partner's outside relationships. They express their feelings, and their partner misconstrues the goal of that communication. Do they just want to express their feelings and receive support and acknowledgment, or are they asking for a change in their partner's behavior or a change in their relationship agreements?" Acting in a reactionary manner to any issue that our partner brings to us is frustratingly common, as is the pain and anger that comes with being told we didn't give our partner what they needed in the moment.

FEELING PATRONIZED

No one likes to be patronized, and even less so when it's coming from a partner. Without meaning to, even very good advice can come across as condescending if it wasn't asked for in the first place. Responding to a partner's pleas for comfort and empathy by giving your own recommendations can send a message that says, "You are not smart enough to figure this out on your own." Or "I know the correct way to solve things, and you don't."

On the flip side, responding to a partner's request for tangible guidance with well-meaning sympathy can send a message that says, "Poor baby. What a pity that you're struggling with that, but I don't have the time or interest to help you out." Which leads us to the next issue . . .

ABANDONMENT AND NEGLECT

So much of communication in relationships is about connection. Even the seemingly innocuous things that your partner says may contain significant appeals for connection: *Listen to me. Care about me. See my pain. Help me out. Comfort me. Take an interest in me. Play with me.* These are sometimes related to "bids for connection," which is a term coined by Drs. John and Julie Gottman for the many small and large ways in which one partner attempts to connect with the other. Inviting a partner to do an activity together, starting a conversation, hinting at an inside joke, or asking for help are some examples of bids for connection (you can find more about bids in the Extra Tools section).

But if you're not aware of those bids, or if you come to a mistaken conclusion about what your partner is seeking, that opportunity for connection is lost and both of you may feel dropped by the other person. When you fail to recognize what your partner is seeking, it can come across as abandonment or neglect: "Sorry, you're on your own here." Or "Your pain and stress don't matter that much to me." Or even "I don't have an interest in what you're feeling." All pretty painful messages to receive from a partner!

NEEDLESS STRESS

All of us have to manage some kind of stress in our lives. There is plenty of it to go around between work, money, family, health, and how you're going to afford your bronze-plated customized miniature for that upcoming Dungeons & Dragons campaign. Cross-purpose communication with a partner is yet another form of stress to add to the pile.

It's stressful to feel like your attempts to fix, comfort, listen, empathize, respond, or soothe are ineffective. It's stressful to ask your partner for advice, comfort, listening, empathy, or soothing only to receive the wrong thing, or to receive nothing at all. Even more so, it's stressful to be caught up in a guessing game, trying to calculate what your partner *really* needs at any given moment.

The "Don't Fix It" Fix-It

Regardless of gender, there are many of us who love to give advice and solve problems. The joy of giving guidance to others can be a wonderful trait, inspiring people to become counselors, therapists, coaches, mentors, teachers, or podcast hosts. But it also has its drawbacks, especially in intimate relationships. "For most of us, it's deeply uncomfortable to see a partner in pain or struggling," shares psychologist Dr. Liz Powell, author of *Building Open Rela-*

tionships. "So when a partner comes to us with a problem, it can be easy to want to find a way to fix the problem, thereby fixing our partner's feelings and our own discomfort as well. We want to jump to the end (Problem solved! Feeling good!) and forget that we can't get there until we spend time on the journey, sitting with our partner and our own feelings."

Research suggests that this is true. A study conducted by Singapore Management University found a correlation between those who are prone to give unsolicited advice and those who seek power and dominance in their lives. Their study found that subconsciously, advice is often given less for the benefit of the recipient and more for the feeling of power it instills in the person giving the advice. The researchers argued that giving advice sometimes creates a power imbalance between two people. Not surprisingly, the study found that women receive unsolicited advice more often than men.

It can be tempting to think that the solution to all of this is simple: only empathize, don't fix! Many relationship experts have come to the same conclusion, going so far as to encourage people (often men) to *always* listen and *never* advise. While refraining from giving unsolicited advice is certainly not the worst approach, we believe that the ability to offer advice and guidance *when it is asked for* can make both parties feel empowered and understand more about each other. From our experience, we've found it is more beneficial for people to learn how to request advice, how to appropriately give advice, and how to be attuned to their partner's requests for advice rather than applying the "Don't fix it!" approach in every circumstance.

Molly and Jake were overall a happy and fun-loving couple, but they kept running into serious communication problems. Their issues would usually rear their ugly heads in the evening, after drinking with friends or when each of them arrived home from work, exhausted from a long and arduous day. Recently, Molly had been complaining about Mark, a mutual friend who worked with Molly and whose behavior was becoming more and more irritating. Though she and Mark got along well, he constantly interrupted her at work, often only giving a cursory "Sorry" before blazing on ahead. Molly was contemplating whether or not she should take the issue to a supervisor, but she felt conflicted. She didn't want to make things awkward in Jake's friendship with Mark. But finally, after a particularly challenging day, she decided to bring up this issue to Jake.

Jake was quiet and methodical and usually spent his time doing the dishes or making dinner while Molly unloaded about whatever was on her mind from the day. In these moments, Jake would try to listen and offer some words of encouragement, but generally he wouldn't say very much during her venting spree. It irked Molly that Jake seemed to take little interest in her dilemma. He seemed totally resistant to helping her come up with a solution.

Jake was taught by his father early on to not give advice to the women he was dating. Advice was reserved for problem-solving with a colleague or a friend, but with the women with whom he was romantically involved, it was better to listen and offer support. He employed these same tactics with Molly because, after all, she never told him to do anything differently. To Molly, Jake's lack of suggestions felt like he wasn't truly engaged in the conversation. She figured, as one of Mark's closest friends, Jake would be the perfect person to help her figure out a way to cope with Mark's behavior. Molly didn't understand why Jake was so nonchalant and unhelpful in trying to find a solution to this issue.

"It seems like you're bored with this conversation. Just forget about it," Molly eventually spit out.

"Jeez, honey, I'm not bored. I swear I'm listening. It's annoying when Mark does that, but he's always been that way. I'm sorry he's upsetting you," Jake said sheepishly. This wasn't the first time Molly had brought up her issues with Mark. Thankfully, after a day or so, she would generally drop the subject and relax a bit.

"I just don't know what to do! I feel like I should bring it up to a supervisor at work, but it's hard doing anything knowing you're such great friends with him, babe. I'm really at a loss here." Molly sighed, hoping Jake would step up with a solution.

"That must be pretty stressful for you. I'm always here whenever you want to vent," Jake offered. He felt proud of how he handled the situation. He hoped that his restraint, listening, and compassion would cheer Molly up without needing to throw his friend under the bus.

Molly, however, was frustrated that Jake wasn't hearing her, and she gave Jake the cold shoulder for the rest of the evening. Molly's anger and dismissal of him made Jake feel like his kind words had backfired. He felt undervalued and unappreciated, two things he very much did not like to feel.

This is yet another example of two people failing to make their needs known or give their partner what they desire from the conversation. Molly deeply wants to feel heard and for Jake to problem-solve with her in the hopes of making her interactions with their mutual friend less challenging. Jake wants to give Molly the reassurance and empathy he thinks she wants. Both have good intentions for themselves and for each other, yet both are frustrated by their partner's inability to give the other what they need. Again, unspecified communication ultimately results in no one getting what they want.

So Meta: Communicating about Communication

After hearing dozens of stories from our clients and listeners, as well as personally going through communication mishaps of our own, the three of us realized how common it is for people to struggle with accurately conveying their needs in a conversation. We sought to find information on how to help our partners, listeners, and ourselves give each other cues and dispel misunderstandings before they even began. That's how we came across the concept of metacommunication.

First coined by English anthropologist Gregory Bateson, metacommunication is essentially "communication about communication." While older definitions of metacommunication focus only on the nonverbal cues we give each other in conversations, such as a sigh, a raise of the eyebrow, or a shrug, modern definitions also include more explicit forms of communication, such as verbal and written. Body language and facial expressions can enable the recipient to gather nuanced data that aids them in understanding more about what is going on during a conversation below the surface. But while nonverbal cues are an essential part of communication, they can also be misinterpreted. To the speaker, the message being relayed might be incredibly apparent and easy to understand. Yet to the listener, in both new and seasoned relationships alike, the meaning of a raised eyebrow or head shake might be misinterpreted. That is why it is important to recognize that metacommunication may also need to be verbal and explicit. Leanne Yau, creator of the nonmonogamy education page Poly Philia, points out an additional reason why direct communication is so important. "As an autistic person, my relationships are founded on making specific requests about our needs and saying exactly what we mean. It's especially difficult for me to interpret indirect statements and social cues, so someone who sulks in silence when they're upset, or who cannot be direct with me about their thoughts and feelings, is a complete deal breaker. When either of us tells the other something, we make sure to specify whether we're doing it just because we want to vent or let them know about it, or if we require them to take a specific action such as offer comfort or help with seeking a solution to a problem."

There are more potential issues with relying exclusively on nonverbal cues for getting one's point across. We were all brought up in different cultures and families of origin who instilled distinct forms of metacommunication within each of us. In the example above, Jake was taught by his family to be patient, stoic, and selective about when to show emotion. To him, he was helping the situation by trying to defuse Molly's anger and remaining restrained during their conversation. It irritated him greatly that Molly didn't appreciate how even-keeled and supportive he was.

Molly, however, came from a family that would regularly show their emotions outwardly through vocal inflections and facial expressions. Her parents and siblings were not afraid to raise their voices during arguments, nor roll their eyes when they found something to be ridiculous. They showed affection just as fiercely with big hugs, shoulder squeezes, and warm embraces. To Molly, Jake's lack of emotion in the face of challenging discussions showed her that he didn't really care about what was bothering her and that he had no meaningful ideas for how to help fix the situation.

It's possible for two people to talk past each other even when they have multiple communication tools at their disposal. Some couples who've had years of experience learning each other's nonverbal cues and who know substantial information about each other's family of origin can pick up on each other's internal meaning with ease. Yet to newer couples, or even long-term partners who have failed to adequately learn what each other's cues mean, relying only on the nonverbal form of metacommunication might exacerbate an issue rather than help.

For clarification, when we discuss metacommunication

throughout this book, we are referring to the more intentional and clear messages that come from direct verbal or written communication. We value clear communication, and we want our metacommunication to be just as clear, rather than relying solely on facial expressions, which are harder to interpret and more difficult to control.

The Triforce of Communication

Once we understood the essential purpose of metacommunication, as well as the pitfalls of nonverbal cues, the three of us sought to take the ideas that we learned from our research and make them universally applicable. We wanted to create a tool that empowered people to communicate easily and effectively, allow each other to be heard, and help them relay what they needed from their partner during any type of conversation. Enter one of the most popular tools that we have ever created: the Triforce of Communication.

The central idea behind the Triforce of Communication is to make it easier to identify and communicate the primary purpose of a given conversation. Our development of this tool came partly from the work of counselor and author Kathy Labriola, the study of metacommunication, and real-world testing by the three of us and our listeners. For this tool to be effective, we realized that it needed to be as simple, straightforward, and easy to understand as possible.

The Triforce of Communication is specifically designed to distill everyday interpersonal communication into three categories, or "Triforces," based on its purpose. Why did we call it the Triforce? Because all three of us are huge fans of the *Legend of Zelda* games. Try as we might to be the cool kids, we can't deny our nerdy roots.

The Triforce of Communication acts as a code that divides communication goals into three categories:

Triforce #1: Sharing and being heard
Triforce #2: Sympathy or celebration
Triforce #3: Advice or decision-making

In the following sections, we will go through each of the three Triforces in detail, describing what it is, why it's used, and some examples of situations where it may be the most useful.

TRIFORCE #1: SHARING AND BEING HEARD

The first Triforce is about sharing information with someone else just to make a thought, feeling, or state of being known. If someone is utilizing Triforce #1, it is not your job to comment or give sympathy or advice unless asked. You may be wondering, "What is the purpose of this Triforce?" For one thing, it can be a very helpful tool to use when initially building a relationship. It can also assist you in understanding your partner's inner world and bring focus to the thoughts and feelings influencing them in any given moment.

Let's look at some examples of Triforce #1:

Sharing a Story

Perhaps the most straightforward example is when the person who is utilizing Triforce #1 shares a story. This could include a story about their childhood, a funny thing that happened during the day, or regaling a young person with tales of old. The important distinction between this Triforce and the others is that communication is generally moving in one direction. The person sharing is relaying information, and the receiver's only job is to listen to that information.

If you're using Triforce #1 when sharing a childhood story, a funny memory from college, or a detailed explanation of why you dislike CrossFit, your goal may simply be to be understood and heard. If, on the other hand, you're sharing a painful memory and you're seeking care and sympathy, you might be seeking Triforce #2 (more on that in the next section). This distinction is significant for you to understand and will allow you to express the type of response you want from your partner.

Letting someone know how you're doing

Let's say you didn't sleep well last night and are having a hard time staying focused today. In a communicative relationship, it can be helpful to give the other person a heads-up: "Hey, I am feeling spacey today. I just wanted to let you know in case I seem distracted. It's not you—I'm just struggling today." This can also be used for feeling down, irritable, or otherwise off from your normal baseline. Again, the important distinction here is that you're just sharing to let the other person know your state of being, and you aren't looking for sympathy or problem-solving.

This can be particularly helpful if you are someone who experiences PTSD, depression, anxiety, or other day-to-day mental or emotional fluctuations, or if you're in a relationship with someone who does. This can also be important for people with chronic pain or illnesses that fluctuate through the day and have a significant impact on their mental state, or while going through periods of heightened stress or recovery. Our traumas and ongoing mental and emotional challenges can often show up unannounced and unexpected, leaving our partners floundering and unsure of how to help. What we need may change from moment to moment, but there can be great freedom in just being able to say, "I felt my anxiety start to get activated this morning. That's why I might seem on edge today. I don't need you to do anything about it or try to fix it, but I just wanted to let you know."

Matter-of-fact scheduling updates
"My Tuesday yoga class got canceled, so I'm going to see if I can schedule a first date for that time" or "I'm going into an intense meeting for the next few hours, so I won't be very communicative for a bit" are examples of important and helpful updates that do not require a specific response from your partner. If your update meant that you would need to reschedule plans with a partner, and thus the two of you would have to work together to find additional time in your busy week, then this would be an example of Triforce #3, problem-solving, which we will cover in a moment.

TRIFORCE #2: SYMPATHY OR CELEBRATION
With the second Triforce, we are not just sharing to be heard; we're communicating because we want our partner to join us and support us emotionally. From sharing a victory at work to mourning the loss of a loved one, having our partner engage with us from a place of emotional care is vital to a healthy relationship. Again, let's look at some examples:

Celebrating a success
You've been working hard on a project and have had some ups and downs, but you've finally made a breakthrough. In these triumphant moments, often the first thing that comes to mind is "I need to tell someone! Who can I call?" The opportunity to celebrate each other's successes is a wonderful experience in a relationship and can cement positive feelings toward one another.

Sharing pain
We all experience the need to let out our feelings and frustrations.

However, this is also one of the most common communication pitfalls for couples. When your partner is desiring Triforce #2, the appropriate response is sympathy and commiseration. Note that a Triforce #2 communication does *not* include advice or suggestions. If we're frustrated about someone at work, we want our partner to take our side, not tell us all the reasons why it's actually our fault. In our experience working with couples, understanding this one distinction and conveying it during a discussion can eliminate a large number of fights.

Seeking encouragement

For many of us, it's difficult to ask for encouragement, but it can be a wonderful way to cultivate intimacy with your partner. After a day of setbacks and frustrations, the ability to say to a partner, "Can you just tell me I'm good at stuff?" or "Can you tell me what you like about me?" can be a lifesaver. In these cases, both partners having a clear sense of what is being requested can make all the difference. When you know your partner wants Triforce #2, then you can offer the support and encouragement they need, rather than wondering if they are secretly criticizing or questioning your affection for them.

TRIFORCE #3: ADVICE OR DECISION-MAKING

The third Triforce is all about getting advice or input from someone else in order to help you problem-solve, collaborate, or make a decision. As we've discussed earlier, advice is not always what is desired or needed, but when it comes Triforce #3, that's exactly what we're going for! Let's look at some real-world examples of Triforce #3 in action:

Deciding what to do together

You and your partner are planning a date night together. They turn to you and say, "I'm having trouble figuring out something fun for us to do tonight." If you respond with, "Wow, that sounds really hard," it's likely to produce frustration. Your partner is probably looking for ideas and brainstorming or help weighing the pros and cons of different options. While that example may seem obvious, there are more subtle ways people can seek Triforce #3. Perhaps the most common example is the living hell that is the "What should we eat tonight?" conversation:

> *"What should we eat tonight?"*
>
> *"I'm fine with whatever. How about you?"*
>
> *"I'm also fine with anything. It's your choice."*
>
> *"Should we cook something at home or go out to eat?"*
>
> *"I'm okay with either."*
>
> *(And so on and so on until somebody faints from low blood sugar.)*

This is a great example of how important it can be to realize that someone is not seeking approval but rather making a call for the listener to step up and collaborate.

Getting help with a personal decision

Another common usage of Triforce #3 is directly asking for help when making a decision. Some examples may include:

> *"I need your help deciding if I should see a therapist."*

"Can you help me pick an outfit for tonight?"

"What do you think I should do about what happened at work today?"

While these examples make it seem obvious that someone is asking for input on their decision, in real life these requests can be more subtle.

"I've been thinking a therapist might help me work through this, but it's also expensive."

"I have no idea what I'm going to wear tonight."

"This situation at work is really stressing me out."

As you can see, it is not always immediately apparent what someone is asking for. If it is unclear what your partner needs at that moment, seek direct confirmation whether they are asking for advice and problem-solving or if they are seeking encouragement and support.

Receiving feedback

There are times when we might seek out someone we trust and respect to get their honest feedback on an idea or a project. This one is especially crucial. Solicited feedback can truly help us grow and improve. Unsolicited feedback, especially from a partner, can feel like painful criticism—often toxic for relationships.

Jase Says

I tend to daydream and brainstorm a lot, and one of the ways that shows up is that I come up with ideas for new podcasts about every other week. Some are silly, some are more serious, but either way I get excited and bring the ideas to Dedeker and Emily to see what they think.

The response is usually along the lines of "That's a fun idea, but let's not do it. Here are X, Y, and Z reasons why it'll be too much work, won't be interesting enough, or is just too darn silly." Fortunately, that kind of response is exactly what I need and have come to expect from them in this situation. It helps me stay focused on the ideas that are really worth pursuing, and on the rare occasion that they approve of the idea, then I can trust that it's good and they aren't just humoring me.

Sometimes, however, I don't want to be practical and just want to have fun fantasizing about a new podcast. I just want them to say, "yes, and" to my ideas and play along rather than just shooting it down right away. In those situations, as soon as they start to respond negatively, I can say, "Just play with me! I know we won't actually do it, but it's a fun idea." Without needing to say specifically that I'm looking for Triforce #2, I'm able to switch the conversation and we can all go along for the ride.

I always encourage people to speak up as soon as they realize they want to switch away from Triforce #3 to Triforce #2. Whether you use those terms or just describe what you're looking for, it can quickly turn a conversation from disappointment and frustration into supportive and silly fun.

Using the Triforce in Real Life

It can be challenging to break free of the bad habits we have built up in previous relationships and easy to rely on the belief that our partner should be able to read our thoughts and innermost feelings. However, with practice and patience, learning to meta-communicate by integrating the Triforce of Communication into everyday conversations can become second nature. A few weeks after learning about the Triforce of Communication, Molly and Jake were able to come back to their previous discussion. Utilizing the Triforce helped both of them get what they wanted and ulti-mately brought their relationship closer together.

Since their last conversation, Molly had been wary of asking for help dealing with the frustrating behavior of Jake's friend Mark. However, after she shared the *Multiamory* episode about the Triforce with Jake, and he took some time to learn about it, she mustered up the courage to finally tell Jake what she needed from him.

"Hey, this is a little difficult for me, but can we try to talk about Mark again? I've been struggling a lot with what's been going on at work recently. I know the two of you are close, and I'd appreciate your help in coming up with a possible solution here," Molly began.

"I'll do my best. Which Triforce are you going for here? Are you looking for my advice?" Jake answered.

"Yeah, that's what I'm going for," Molly said. "I know I've already talked to you a little about this over the last few weeks. He constantly interrupts me when we're in meetings together at work, and he even does it sometimes when you and I are hanging out with him together. He sometimes apologizes but doesn't really do anything to fix it, and it's getting on my nerves. I don't think he's a bad guy, but something needs to change. I don't want to make things weird between us or make your friendship with him uncomfortable. I am just not sure how to proceed here."

"I have noticed him doing that before," Jake admitted. "But it seems like we're all usually able to laugh it off, so I never thought about it much. I can understand how that could be even more frustrating having to deal with it at work, too. If it were me, I would just talk to him directly about it. He can dominate conversations without thinking, but knowing him, he also takes feedback about that stuff pretty well. If he knew that this was bothering you, I'm sure he would want to make it right. Do you feel okay doing that or is there something that I can do to help?" he asked.

"Honestly, you're his best friend, and I think you could also speak up in some way. When we're all hanging out together, I don't want to bring down the mood. But if I know that you are keeping an eye out for that and backing me up, I think I'd feel a lot more at ease," Molly offered.

"I can definitely do that. We'll figure this out together," said Jake.

This is a great example of two people using Triforce #3 to help make their needs known. Molly and Jake's conversation had a significantly different outcome when they employed the Triforce than when they could only guess and assume what they needed from one another. First, Molly set up the situation by relaying to Jake that she values his opinion and that she feels like he is the one person who could help her most effectively with this issue. She let Jake know from her statement that she wants advice on the situation, and that she wants his help in problem-solving a way toward a solution.

Jake stepped up to the plate immediately and clarified that what she's looking for is advice. Even though Jake specifically referenced the Triforce as a shorthand, it's possible for this conversation to turn out the same way even if he hadn't used that specific terminology. Further on in the conversation, after hearing the particulars of Mark's behavior, Jake not only offered the advice she requested, but took a further step to ask what else he could do to help her in this scenario. This is a fantastic example of taking the more abstract musings of a conversation and turning them into actionable, collaborative steps the couple can take to achieve their goals.

Finally, by the conclusion of their conversation, the two have created an opportunity for more intimacy by acknowledging that each of them made the other feel heard and loved, and that they were able to fulfill what their partner asked of them. This is the ultimate goal of the Triforce—to give you and your partner a greater understanding of each other and the unique ways in which you each communicate. This knowledge will allow you more time to enjoy the benefits of being in a relationship with one another and diminish potential arguments that might occur due to a misunderstanding of each other's personal metacommunication style.

One-sided Metacommunication

This is great and all, you may be thinking. *But now I have to onboard everyone in my life with this nerdy communication tool in order for it to work.*

As much as we love shoving our geeky communication tools in other people's faces, it's not necessary for people to know about the Triforce of Communication in order for it to be effective. As long as at least one party is knowledgeable in the ways of the Triforce, it can be both collaborative and unilateral. To see an example of using the Triforce one-sided, we can see how Taylor and Sebastian managed to resolve their conflict over Sebastian's new work schedule.

After their frustrating conversation, Taylor learned about the Triforce of Communication from the *Multiamory* podcast.

Thinking back on his miscommunication with Sebastian and knowing that he often has the urge to solve problems, Taylor was able to recognize that Seb assumed he was asking for Triforce #3 when Taylor really just wanted the comfort and sympathy of Triforce #2. Taylor recognized that there probably weren't specific changes Sebastian needed to make, and he didn't want to add any additional stress to his plate. But, despite his understanding of the hardships Seb was facing in the new job, he felt it was important to remind Sebastian of his needs and ask for some compassion and tenderness. Taylor was feeling better after learning the reasons behind their earlier communication breakdown, but he was also cautious that Sebastian might still be upset and think he wanted him to change something about his job commitments. He waited to bring it up until they were both in a more relaxed state of mind on the weekend, as opposed to after Seb was already tired from work, and he did it in a more thoughtful and pragmatic way.

"Listen, there's something that's been on my mind for a while. I want you to know that even though I'm saying this, you don't need to fix a problem or change anything that you are doing. I just want you to understand how I am feeling," began Taylor.

"Okay," said Sebastian hesitantly. "What is it?"

"I'm happy for you getting this job, but lately I've been feeling kind of sad and missing you a lot. It's been hard not seeing each other as frequently as we used to. I recognize that there are things I can do to combat those feelings, and I think overall I would just love a little extra sweetness and connection while we're both getting used to this transition. Does that make sense?" he said.

"We've already been over this!" Seb immediately responded. "I said I'm not going to do any more overtime this week! Doesn't that help you feel any better? Or do you need me to call in sick from work or something?"

"No, not at all. You've already done a lot, and I'm proud to be here to support you while you're taking on all this new responsibility. I don't need you to make any changes or try to fix this. I know it helps you to vent and share your frustrations with work in the evenings, and I'm happy to support you with that. I just want to be able to share my frustration, too. Not so you can fix it, but because we're a team together and I miss spending as much quality time with you."

"I think I can handle that," Sebastian replied, slowly relaxing his shoulders and beginning to understand what Taylor was asking. "I appreciate knowing how you're feeling. I really have been missing you a lot lately, too. It makes sense that you'd be feeling neglected in the midst of all this. I'd be having a hard time, too, if the tables were turned. Can I give you a hug?"

"I would love that." Taylor smiled as Seb scooped him up in his arms. "Even if we don't have as much free time together, I like getting to connect with you. I'd love it if maybe we could spend some time tonight away from the TV to cuddle, and maybe next weekend we could do something special, just the two of us? I'd love the opportunity to connect in a meaningful way."

Sebastian was not aware of the Triforce of Communication, but he was able to give Taylor the Triforce #2 that he wanted. Taylor recognized that he needed to make it clear from the beginning of their conversation that he didn't want Sebastian to fix how he was feeling. Taylor also let him know that while he would appreciate extra empathy and support from Seb, he was also responsible for doing his own work when it came to dealing with his emotions. Finally, he suggested some ways in which the two of them could connect with one another immediately and in the near future. Sebastian then felt empowered and excited to express love and give Taylor the empathy and understanding that he needed.

Breaking old miscommunication patterns can be difficult,

but by learning the ways in which communication has gotten confused in the past and taking proactive steps to clarify what you are seeking, you can adjust those habits and gradually improve the quality of your conversations. From overnight transformations to longer-term changes to well-worn routines, we continue to be amazed and impressed with the positive impact that this relatively simple tool has had on our audience's lives.

Troubleshooting

I want to try this, but what if my partner isn't on board?
If you're reading this book, we're assuming that you have some interest in communication hacks and other relationship geekery. Your partner, however, may not. But never fear! The Triforce of Communication can still be helpful.

If you and your partner have been able to acknowledge that you've run into conflict because of communication at cross-purposes, that is already a huge first step. Get creative and come up with a shorthand that works for both of you. You can come up with a code word or phrase that either person can use to call it out and change course in the moment: "Looks like we're doing our usual song and dance. Let's reset. What do you need from me right now?" Personally, we love these kinds of shorthand phrases or code words because of how easy they can be to use, even in challenging situations (we cover Microscripts in depth in Chapter 4).

As we spoke about previously, you can also use the Triforce as a unilateral guide for yourself to get better at advocating for what you need as well as asking your partner for what they need. Even without using the shorthand of T1, T2, T3, you can spell things out more explicitly:

> *"I appreciate the advice, but I think right now I just want you to hold me and reassure me that everything is going to be okay."*

> *"If you like, I can share with you how I've handled a situation like this in the past, or I can just listen while you vent. Does one of those sound better to you right now?"*

I keep defaulting to my old habit of giving advice.
By the time many of us are in our first adult relationships, we've had several years of exposure to one particular communication style— usually that of our parents, family of origin, or cultural background. Dedeker grew up in an extremely pragmatic family, where feelings of sadness or loneliness weren't addressed with listening, empathy, or comfort but were treated as problems to be solved. She then went on to become a relationship coach and consultant, which means several years of a deeply worn neural pathway that favors doling out advice and solutions whether they are asked for or not (she is eternally grateful for her patient partners).

These kinds of neural pathways can take a lot of repetition to reforge. Being able to notice the moment you fall back into old habits is key, combined with the ability to pivot and reset in the moment:

> *"Oops, I realize that I jumped straight into T3 even though you didn't ask for it. I'm sorry about that. What are you looking for at this moment?"*

> *"I realize that I'm giving you my opinion without checking in with you first. Is it better if I switch gears?"*

And remember, if your partner points out that you're giving a

63

different Triforce than what they asked for, do whatever it takes to accept it *gracefully* and adjust accordingly.

What if I don't know which Triforce to ask for?
That's totally normal and okay! We don't always have a clear understanding of what we need, especially in moments that feel emotional, chaotic, or confusing. We recommend starting out by being honest with the other person about feeling unclear:

> *"I've had some money troubles on my mind today. I want to talk it out, but I'm not entirely sure what I'm looking for here. Can I just start out with you listening and then figure it out from there?"*

As you're communicating, take time to check in with your feelings. Does it feel good to just be able to talk while your partner listens? Are you feeling a sense of disappointment that your partner isn't responding in a particular way? Be on the lookout for little clues letting you know what's working and what isn't.

I thought I wanted some advice and asked for T3, but then I started feeling upset and defensive while listening to my partner's advice.
Sometimes we don't always have the most accurate sense of what we need in the moment. If you asked for a particular Triforce, only to find that you're feeling upset, dissatisfied, or misunderstood, that may be a sign that it's time to change course. The good news is that it's possible to change your mind, pivot, and ask for what you need.

> *"I know I asked for your advice, but I'm realizing that I may actually just want some empathy."*

"I appreciate you comforting and supporting me through this, but I think I need to consider solutions. Can I also get your take on what you would do in this situation?"

Homework

With most things in life, it is easier to learn and practice a skill when the stakes are low. Then, in the heat of the moment, you'll have some experience and a foundation for using the skills when they really count. We recommend this approach when working through this and the subsequent homework assignments we've laid out for you in the upcoming chapters.

With a friend or romantic partner, try this exercise to get in the habit of using the Triforce. It's okay if it seems silly at first. In fact, silliness actually helps ideas stick in your brain and can make them not feel so daunting during the times when they really matter.

Start with one person taking the role of Partner One and the other taking the role of Partner Two. Go through the steps and then switch roles and try again.

1. Partner One picks a story from their day to share with Partner Two. It could be something silly, mundane, stressful, disappointing, exciting, fun, or anything else (for this exercise, start with something easy—ideally an event that wasn't too upsetting).

2. After Partner One is finished sharing, Partner Two asks them what Triforce they are looking for (sharing, support/ celebration, or advice/problem-solving).

3. Partner One picks a Triforce, and Partner Two then tries to give a response that fits.

4. Next, Partner One will say, "Actually, I would appreciate something else." Partner One will pick a different Triforce this time.

5. Partner Two will try to give a separate response (to the same story) that fits the new Triforce.

6. Finally, Partner One will ask for the last Triforce, and Partner Two attempts to give yet another response that fits.

Now switch roles and try it again. Being silly with this exercise can actually help make the contrasts between the individual Triforces more apparent. There's no need to take the exercise too seriously!

Takeaways

- Metacommunication is communicating *about* your communication. For the purposes of this book, we mean verbal, written, or other explicit communication.

- The Triforce is a tool for dividing all communication into three categories:
  - O Triforce 1—Sharing and Connecting
  - O Triforce 2—Support or Celebration
  - O Triforce 3—Advice or Problem-Solving

- Telling your partner what you need from an interaction not only helps you get what you want but it makes it easier for them to give it to you.

- If you aren't sure what someone needs from you, it's okay to ask.

- The more you communicate using the Triforce, the more easily you will learn to identify what others need.

For more information, check out *Multiamory* Episode 83, The Triforce of Communications and Episode 159, "The Triforce of Communication: DLC Expansion Pack."

The Triforce of Communication Cheat Sheet

TRIFORCE	EXAMPLE DIALOGUE
TRIFORCE #1, T1 Sharing a story, building connection, status updates	Person A: I'm gonna tell you the story of the hilarious Google Calendar mishap I had with my partners last week. Person B: *explodes into LOLs* Person A + B: *high-fives*

TRIFORCE	EXAMPLE DIALOGUE
TRIFORCE #2, T2 Seeking support, acknowledgment, empathy, encouragement	Person A: I came out of the closet to my mother, and she reacted badly. I could really use some support right now. Person B: I'm sorry to hear that you're having a hard time. I had a similar experience when I came out to my mother, and I know it can really suck. You'll make it through this one! Person A: I feel listened to and vali-dated. Thank you. Person A + B: *high-fives*

TRIFORCE	EXAMPLE DIALOGUE
TRIFORCE #3, T3 Solving a problem or seeking advice, collaboration, team-work	Person A: My partner is going out on a first date tonight, and I'm having a rough time with it because I'll be home alone. I could use some advice and suggestions on how to get through this. Person B: The last time I was the one left home alone, I just went out for a run and listened to my favorite podcast. It really helped me get my mind off it. Would something like that be helpful to you? Person A: Actually, yes, I think I'll try that. Thanks for the suggestion! Person A + B: *high-fives*

CHAPTER 3 | **Spewers and Chewers:** Be Proactive About Your Processing Style

E rika and Kaori had been dating for a couple years when they started contemplating moving in together. Erika's lease was ending soon, and they were trying to decide if she should renew it for another year, move into Kaori's place, or look for a new apartment together. They were both nervous and excited about the big decision, but over the course of discussing the pros and cons, frustration began to emerge.

Kaori liked to think out loud, brainstorm, and bounce ideas off Erika. "If we got a new place together, we'd have to wait a few months until my lease ends, but we could move your stuff in here temporarily until then. Though, maybe if your stuff was here, you'd rather unpack and settle in. So maybe we could just start by living here together for a while instead of immediately looking for a new place. I know you like your current apartment, too, but you seemed more interested in living in this part of town since it's closer to your new job. What do you think?"

Erika sat there sheepishly for a moment, not knowing what to say. "Yeah, that's all true. I just don't know. I need to think about it." This seemed reasonable to her, but Kaori started to get frustrated.

"Yeah, I know we need to think about it. That's what I'm trying to do. There are a lot of options, and I want to be sure that we're making a decision that feels right for you and feels right for our relationship. I want to be sure you aren't feeling pressured or anything, either." Kaori was starting to worry that Erika's lack of interest in this discussion meant she was getting cold feet about living together—and maybe even about being in the relationship at all.

Erika was just desperate to get her thoughts in order. "Yeah, I appreciate that. I'll keep thinking about it and let you know."

Kaori was beginning to fear there was a reason Erika didn't want to discuss the prospect of moving in with her. Was it too soon? Was she being too pushy about this? "All right, let's just not even worry about this now. I mean, you like your place a lot, and it's nice to visit each other, so maybe it would be better to keep our separate places."

Erika's eyes began to well up as Kaori seemingly bailed on the plan to live together. "Okay . . . if that's what you want, then I'll just have to figure something out to somehow afford this neighborhood or keep my apartment and do this commute every day," she mumbled between tears.

"Hey, what's going on, sweetie? I just want to know what feels good for you!" Kaori insisted, caught off guard.

"But you just said that you think it's better if we didn't live together! You literally just said it. I don't want you to invite me here out of pity or obligation."

As Erika continued to sob, Kaori looked around with eyes wide, trying to understand what just happened. How had this conversation become an occasion for tears instead of excitement about building a future together?

Spewers and Chewers: An Introduction

It's not uncommon to start out a discussion feeling like you and your partner are on the same team, only for it to morph into an unexpected argument. With Erika and Kaori, a misunderstanding seemed to emerge out of nowhere and caused feelings of hurt, even though that was not the intention of either woman. Personal communication styles are complex and unique, and often it's challenging to remember that our friends, family members, and partners don't always share the same communication patterns that we do. After hearing hundreds of listener and client stories, we've noticed a particular type of communication breakdown that occurs due to the different ways people process and communicate with one another about their thinking.

In the example above, these two women are polar opposites when it comes to their communication styles. Erika is an internal processor, which in *Multiamory*-speak is known as a "Chewer." Kaori is an external processor, otherwise known as a "Spewer." When two people have different processing methods and fail to recognize or learn to work with those fundamental differences, it can lead to miscommunication, hurt feelings, frustration, and resentment. In fact, Dedeker and Jase had a similar interaction to Kaori and Erika when Dedeker made a snap decision to become a digital nomad and travel the world while working on her first book. They were trying to figure out how to maintain their relationship, weighing up decisions about if or when Jase might travel with her, or when she might come back to the US for visits. It was a difficult discussion, largely because Jase and Dedeker each fall on opposite ends of the spectrum when it comes to chewing and spewing.

Jase and Emily are Spewers—they love to talk through problems before every detail is ironed out or solidified. Their ideas evolve and grow as they discuss an issue out loud. Dedeker, on the other hand, is a bona fide Chewer. She will internally work

73

through problems on her own before bringing more fully formed ideas to a conversation. There was a lot of strife at *Multiamory* production meetings until we figured this out! Both communication processing styles have distinct sets of strengths as well as complexities and challenges for both the processor and the recipient. But, before we break down each category, it's important to address the purpose of using these labels.

An Interlude on Labels

You may have heard the common phrases "I'm a dog person" or "I'm very type A." Of course, there is the classic "I'm an introvert" or "I'm an extrovert." In recent years, there has been an explosion of granular labels for a beautiful variety of gender identities, sexual orientations, relationship practices, and more. More complex and nuanced classifications have become all the rage, and countless online quizzes can tell you things like your Myers-Briggs personality type, what your zodiac sign says about you, and how your attachment style can alter and shape your relationships. So what's the deal with all these labels? Do labels help us, or do they trap us in a box?

On the positive end, labels can help provide a sense of identity, allow us to understand more about the complexities of how our brains and bodies work, or help us feel connected to others like us. In essence, labels can help make us feel like we aren't alone in the world. However, labels can also heighten a sense of otherness between ourselves and those who are different from us. Labels have the potential to contribute to polarization, fear, and distrust. They can encourage negative associations with a person or group of people based on the information we've gleaned from our culture about what someone with that label must be like. While it is important to acknowledge and honor our own individual labels, we must also work to not fall into the trap of characterizing or stigmatizing others. The purpose of labels is not to determine what is good or bad, but simply to provide an identifying tool to aid better understanding of ourselves and one another.

Keep this knowledge in mind as you continue to learn more about internal and external processing. While certain Spewers and Chewers may find that our descriptions of each communication style resonate with their personal experience, others may realize that they are a blend of both styles, or that they operate in a slightly different way from what we have described. The important thing is to spend time getting curious and to learn about the unique way you communicate. Be specific with your partners about your needs and desires when you discuss with them the most effective ways in which they can communicate with you. Poly Philia creator Leanne Yau says, "Just because someone loves and cares about you, it doesn't necessarily mean they're so attuned to you that they can read your mind. More often than not, our partners have different boundaries, priorities, and ways of handling various situations, and some of them may surprise you if you don't ask!" The goal in learning about our partner's communication style is to cultivate ways in which each of you can work together to build understanding, respect, and appreciation for all the unique things that make you . . . well, you!

Are You a Chewer or a Spewer?

If you are unaware of your own processing style, it can limit your ability to empathize and relate to people who are on the other end of the spectrum. While it can take a little extra work to connect to a partner whose chewy or spewy style is different from your own, the relationship benefits are ultimately immense. Step one is just understanding that these variations exist. For the three of us, simply identifying that processing styles may feel different from person to person was a huge step toward having more understanding, patience, and empathy for one another.

Step two is evaluating where you personally fall on the Spew/Chew continuum. You may not fall distinctively into one category or the other, but chances are good that there is one side of the spectrum you are more likely to lean toward. Knowing which direction you lean can unlock crucial understanding for improving your communication. When Jase and Dedeker realized that he is a Spewer and she is a Chewer, it took away much of the guilt and shame around past conflicts. They learned that much of it was due to their different ways of processing thoughts and feelings, rather than a deeper incompatibility or a lack of caring for one another.

So which one are you? We'll start with what it's like to be a Chewer. Read these statements and think about how much you resonate with them. Do they clearly reflect your experience? Can you relate to some or all of them? Do any of them seem like a foreign concept? Or do they sound like a description of someone you know? All of these questions are useful to help you understand what it means to be a Chewer and whether or not you might be one yourself.

You might be a Chewer if . . .

- When faced with a dilemma or emotional decision, you need time alone to process your thoughts. Journaling or meditation are often helpful ways of doing this.

- You don't like having to state your opinion or feelings until they are fully formed.

- When you do state a decision, it's final and not likely to be up for further discussion.

- You are hesitant to share your thoughts while in the midst of processing unless you feel very safe.

- Before a meeting or presentation, you prefer lots of prep time to organize your thoughts.

- You form complete thoughts in your head before saying them out loud.

- You choose your words carefully and deliberately.

- Others sometimes accuse you of being unemotional, rigid, or withdrawn.

- During a heated discussion, you feel a need to take a time-out to process your thoughts.

Now let's take a look at Spewers. Read these next statements and evaluate how they resonate with you. Do these sound like you? Do they sound like someone you know?

You might be a Spewer if . . .

- When faced with a dilemma or emotional decision, you want to seek out a trusted friend to listen while you talk it out.

- You feel trapped or stuck if you can't find anyone to talk to about a decision or your feelings.

- When you are talking through your feelings, you may say things that you don't actually believe or agree with while trying to work something out.

- You find it hard to keep your thoughts and feelings inside and would prefer to share them out loud to help understand them.

- You love brainstorming and sharing ideas with others.

- It's hard to know what you truly believe until you've said it out loud and evaluated how you feel about it.

- You may talk out loud to process even if nobody is around to hear you.

- Free-association writing may be helpful as a way to process your thoughts.

After looking at the lists above, you might immediately know if you are a Chewer or a Spewer. Or you might identify with points from either side. Remember that this is a spectrum, not a binary. The important thing to recognize is that these processing and communication traits exist and manifest in a variety of unique ways in different people. It may be difficult to imagine what life is like for someone whose style is different from your own, but hopefully gaining knowledge of how the other side operates can be a starting point for increased empathy.

SPEWERS V. CHEWERS: WHO WOULD WIN?

Good news: there is nothing wrong with the way that you process! There is also nothing wrong with the way your partner processes.

Hold on, Multiamory, you might say. It's frustrating that my partner is so quiet/conflict avoidant/shut down/vocal/rambly/worked up/[insert your own word here]. There's gotta be something to fix.

We all have our bad communication habits. Every one of us has moments of speaking to those close to us in harsh and unkind ways. All of us have either avoided a dialogue in order to feel safe and comfortable, or we've pushed a dialogue on someone else who wasn't ready to talk. Arguably, these are all fixable problems. However, the way that we each inherently process information may not be "fixable," and that can cause friction.

In the next chapter, we'll talk more about using our brain's natural plasticity to adjust and grow out of bad communication habits. If you're a Spewer, you might consider "trying on" some Chewer practices to see how they feel. If you're a Chewer, you might consider finding a safe person to experiment with some spewing and see how it feels. But, if you're not interested in changing the way that you process, that's also okay.

Rather than getting down on yourself or your partner for not processing the way you'd like, start where you are at this moment. Embrace the way your brain and heart work, then look for ways to help that jell with the people who are close to you with as much kindness and ease as possible.

Beware the Dark Side

Each style comes with its own unfortunate drawbacks. These are the areas where we've seen an individual's processing style cause misunderstanding, misattunement, and hurt feelings all around. Do any of the following pitfalls ring true for you or your experience of someone else?

FOR CHEWERS

- As a Chewer, you may find that your thinking can end up limited or narrow because you are processing all on your own.

- You may experience frustration if asked to weigh in on something before having time to think it through, and you may act out of that frustration.

- Others may be offended by your silence or lack of immediate response when presented with information.

- You may need lots of unstructured time throughout the day to process your thoughts and work through problems on your own.

- Collaboration on problem-solving can be challenging if you haven't had time to work out solutions in advance or if others are more likely to spew than chew.

FOR SPEWERS

- Others may be confused when you change your mind, thinking that you already came to a final decision while you were working through possibilities out loud.

- Others may see your external processing as being wishy-washy or inconsistent.

- Others may be hurt by something you said while you were processing if they believed it to be a fully formed opinion.

- People in your life may feel overwhelmed by your words, find you difficult to follow, or need to take a break from the conversation when you are externally processing your thoughts or feelings.

Myths and Misconceptions

When we look at the chewing-spewing spectrum, some recurring themes emerge. As you go farther along the chewer side of the spectrum, there are more behaviors where energy moves *inward*. At the spewer end, there are more behaviors where energy moves *outward*. This pairing can bring to mind other spectrums of personality, identity, or attachment style. However, it's important that we don't automatically jump to conclusions. Here are some common myths and misconceptions about the ways in which being a Spewer or Chewer may inform your personality, identity, or even attachment style:

Myth #1: Men are always Chewers. Women are always Spewers.
It's been long held as fact within pop psychology that processing styles run along strict gender lines. The most common assumption is that people socialized as men are more likely to be internal processors, while people socialized as women tend to be external processors (to be more accurate, people don't usually include caveats for socialization. This assumption is often presented as an ironclad reality: men and women are just born this way). John Gray, author of the 1992 classic *Men Are From Mars, Women Are From Venus,* calls a man's internal processing and desire to pull away "Cave Time," and he argues that, "As a woman, learning how to make peace with Cave Time is one of the most important things you can do to set yourself up for long-term happiness in your relationship."

Truthfully, we think that's a load of crap. There are indeed many social factors that encourage men to be stoic and silent and encourage women to connect and converse. However, there are also plenty of forces that push in the opposite direction, creating copious space for men to speak and pontificate and punishing women for talking too much or too loudly or for speaking up at all. In addition, these stereotypes erase people who don't fit into a neat category within a gender binary. Just as much of the relationship research out there primarily focuses on white, heterosexual, cisgender relationships, so do many popular self-help books. There are plenty of Spewers and Chewers out there who don't fall along traditional gender lines (Jase and Dedeker are brilliant examples).

Myth #2: Chewers are always introverted. Spewers are always extroverted.
Another common myth about internal and external processors is that those who process internally are automatically introverts,

and those who process externally must clearly be extroverts. Introverts are recharged by quiet alone time, while extroverts are refueled by groups of people in social settings. This isn't to say that introverts don't like social situations. In fact, an introvert may love being around a large group of people, but their "batteries" are recharged by having some space and time for themselves. Conversely, an extrovert might occasionally wish to spend quiet time alone, but they also thrive on exciting moments where they can be the center of attention for an evening. One's communication style does not automatically set the stage for how they will feel most rejuvenated. An extroverted Chewer might find that having other people around while they chew helps them feel more stable or supported. An introverted Spewer might only feel comfortable spewing to a close friend within the privacy of their own home.

Myth #3: Chewers always have an avoidant attachment style. Spewers always have an anxious attachment style.
Processing styles are generally unrelated to attachment styles (for a quick rundown of attachment styles, check out the section on attachment theory in the Extra Tools section). Someone who has an avoidant attachment style may just as easily be a Spewer or a Chewer, and someone with secure or insecure attachment could also fall into either category. However, a person's attachment style can certainly influence the way in which they chew or spew, which can allow for a more nuanced understanding of yourself or your partner. An avoidant-attached Spewer may use their external processing style to protect themselves from getting hurt by avoiding any full declarations of their feelings or desires. An avoidant Chewer may have learned that they are safest when keeping more of their thoughts to themselves and therefore choose to only share them once they have weighed all the pros and cons. Meanwhile,

an anxious-attached Chewer may have learned that their partners respond positively when they keep their inner mental ruminations to themselves. Conversely, an anxious-attached Spewer may have adapted to share their evolving feelings in real time as a way to get closer to a partner, in addition to picking up on cues that indicate their partner's feelings.

New Understanding

In the weeks after their unfortunate conversational disaster regarding the decision to live together or not, Kaori and Erika were fortunate to come across the *Multiamory* podcast episode on Chewers and Spewers (Episode 264). Kaori listened to the episode first and suddenly felt like she was able to pick up the pieces of their conversation and reassemble them into something that made sense. She immediately shared the information with Erika, and together they began to see many more of their past conflicts and miscommunications in a new light. When Kaori exclaimed to Erika that she was probably a Spewer, Erika laughed out loud at how obvious that was. Similarly, neither of them hesitated to recognize Erika's Chewiness.

A few days later, Kaori came to Erika, her head full of thoughts and possibilities about their living situation. "Babe, I've been thinking a lot about our options and wanted to take a bit to spew some thoughts at you. It's all just kind of in-progress thinking, and nothing is final or set in stone. It'll just help me to say it out loud."

Erika agreed, and Kaori took some time to ramble about her ideas, new possibilities, the pros and cons of different choices, her fears, and her excitement. There were moments when Erika felt herself tune out at the onslaught of words, but instead of getting overwhelmed, she was able to remind herself that she didn't need to take in or understand everything. It reminded her of the experience of looking at an Impressionist painting and letting it wash over her rather than trying to make out each individual item in the picture.

"Okay, I hope that all makes sense and that we can ultimately come to a good decision together. If you're able, I'd love to get any insights into how you're feeling about all this," Kaori finished.

Erika took a moment. "I've also been thinking about this a lot. I do like the idea of living with you, but it's also a big decision, and I know I've got some of my own baggage around it to work out. Even if we don't move in together right away, I'm still interested in doing that at some point. I'm also excited about the idea of just jumping in and doing it now, but I don't feel like I can pin down my thoughts any further. Is it all right to just know that I'm also thinking about it and give me some time to keep processing my feelings?"

"Of course." Kaori smiled. "I feel ridiculous, but it means a lot just to know you are thinking about it and not just avoiding it. Do you have any sense of when you might be able to share the results of your chewing?"

"Maybe at dinner on Saturday? I should have some time later this week, and I can prioritize getting my thoughts in order. I know you've been anxious to start making some decisions, so I will try to do as much processing as I can by then. I appreciate you giving me the time, and I'm glad to know that you don't expect me to make sense of all the thoughts you spew at me sometimes." Erika laughed.

Kaori couldn't help but laugh, too. "I don't even understand all the stuff that comes out of my mouth while I'm working through something! It means a lot to me when you do share what's going on in your head with me, even if they aren't final thoughts yet. It helps me to have a sense of where you're coming from while you're still working through it."

Erika and Kaori resolved their misunderstanding by using many of the metacommunication tactics that we discussed in the previous chapter. The two women were thoughtful about how they approached this talk and set themselves up for success by giving some time and space away from the heightened emotions of their tiff. Even though it was challenging for Kaori, the Spewer of the relationship, to pause the conversation prematurely, she decided to try and honor Erika's request to save the discussion for later. Similarly, Erika was able to remind herself that it was safe to share some thoughts that weren't fully formed while still being clear that she needed more time before making a final decision.

The women were also able to talk specifically about how each of them uniquely processed their thoughts and feelings. Clear and honest discussions that are objective and direct are a great place to start when talking to your partner about your individual communication style. Additionally, they considered possible actions to help one another in times of need. Some of these solutions weren't immediately intuitive to the way in which each of them process, but they tried to find behaviors that would honor their partner's wants, needs, and preferences.

Spewers and Chewers in Real Life

In the spirit of embracing our differences and finding practical ways to communicate and apply this newfound knowledge, here are some suggestions for using your Spewer or Chewer nature to enhance your communication and reduce friction with others.

IF YOU'RE A SPEWER . . .

Do a pre-spew
Your partner just dropped some news on you, and already you are full of thoughts, opinions, questions, concerns, and feelings. Before launching into a full-force spew, consider pausing and finding a place or person to prespew to.

You're just trying to turn me into a Chewer!

Fear not, dear reader! On the contrary, we encourage you to start spewing right away, *just not directly at your partner.* Jumpstart that external processing by reaching out to your support network. Find a trusted friend or therapist. If that's not practical at the moment, do a big writing dump into a journal or bust out the colored pencils and start drawing. What you're trying to do here is lessen the impact of the tidal wave on your partner without sacrificing the way that you process. By the time you're ready to dialogue with your partner, you may still need to externally process, but hopefully in a way that carries less emotional weight. A less overwhelmed partner is a partner who can better listen and hold space.

Ask ahead of time if it's okay to spew
Sprinkling in just a tiny bit of consideration and metacommunication can do wonders. This could be something as simple as, "I have a lot on my mind about XYZ, and I would appreciate having a listening ear. Is now a good time for me to talk some things out?" Bonus points if you use the Triforce from Chapter 2 to clarify exactly what you're seeking. Even more bonus points if this request is presented in a way where the other person feels safe to say no.

Check in frequently

Do your best to maintain an awareness of the listener while you're spewing. Depending on your partner's personality, they may not be the first one to speak up when feeling overwhelmed or confused. It doesn't have to be formal. Something as simple as "Is this making sense?" or "Is it okay for me to continue, or should we take a little break?" should suffice.

Set a timer

If you know you are a copious Spewer and it's having a negative effect on your discussions, set a timer for yourself. This is going to be successful if *you* are choosing to set a timer for *yourself*. If you're a partner of a Spewer trying to force a time limit, it's probably not going to go down well. Instead, try one of the suggestions below.

IF YOU'RE A CHEWER . . .

Overcommunicate what you need

Your partner just dropped some news on you, and already you are full of thoughts, opinions, questions, concerns, and feelings. It's a lot, and you know you need to retreat and take some time to sort through it all. Before bailing on the conversation, consider taking some time to overcommunicate to your partner about what you need.

> *You're just trying to turn me into a Spewer!*

Fear not, dear reader! On the contrary, we encourage you to chew to your heart's content, *but with consideration for bringing your partner up to speed*. This means including as much detail as you can about your chewing plan. Your chewing plan may include communicating the following:

"I'm going to take X amount of time to chew on this."

"I am going to go to X location to chew on this."

"I will approach you when I have thoroughly chewed" or *"Can you please ask me about this again after X amount of time?"*

"I'd like some alone time while I'm chewing on this" or *"I'm okay to talk about other things and maintain connection in the meantime."*

A common criticism of Chewers is that their partners feel abandoned, shut out, or left in the dark when they retreat to process. By communicating as much detail as you possibly can, it helps to minimize feelings of rupture and anxiety.

Set some time limits
As part of overcommunicating your chewing plan, get specific about a time frame. Unnecessary anxiety can occur when one person takes a break from a conversation without giving any indication of when or if they'll be coming back to continue the dialogue. This may be trickier than it sounds, however. If you're juggling a million different thoughts, feelings, and questions, it can be difficult to drum up the mental resources to make a decision about how long you'll need to sift through it all. Toss in a little bit of activation and anger, and it gets really tempting to make a dramatic exit, leaving your partner regretful and pining for the mysterious hour of your return (we have all been there).

We recommend negotiating some amount of time between twenty minutes on the low end and twenty-four hours on the high end. In an ideal world, this would be more than enough time to regulate emotions, get your thoughts in order, and feel prepared to open up the topic again with your partner. In the real world, there can be any number of obstacles to this, such as work schedules, parenting responsibilities, unexpected illness, bouts of depression, a flat tire, and more. If twenty-four hours have passed and you find yourself needing more processing time, make the effort to check in with your partner. Proactively express that you are still aware of the question or topic at hand and indicate how much more time you'd like.

Make an effort to express connection and affection

This one requires you to build a very important skill—the ability to be kind and courteous to your partner even when you're upset, overwhelmed, or in need of solo time. It may seem like hitting the EJECT button on an emotionally tense conversation as soon as possible is the key to minimizing damage, and a lot of Chewers opt for this tactic. As much as we advocate for taking pauses and advocating for what you need, it will all go to waste if the effect it leaves on your partner is one of being cut off, deserted, and hurt.

This skill acts like a muscle; it gets easier and more natural the more you train it and flex it. Even if you're leaving the conversation to chew, express to your partner that you are still there for them in a way that lands for them. This doesn't have to be effusive or phony. Gentle, nonaggressive honesty combined with clarity about when you'll be back is a good route to take: "I'm having a lot of thoughts and feelings come up right now, and I need a little bit of time to get my thoughts in order. I'm going to take a walk, and I will be back in half an hour."

IF YOUR PARTNER IS A SPEWER . . .

Use metacommunication to clarify what's needed
Triforce of Communication to the rescue! Ask your partner what they are looking for and ask often! It's always a good time to clarify, whether that's before, during, or after your beloved Spewer's spiel. This is going to help you to know what kind of listening to provide. Having a clear sense of direction will help keep you grounded as your partner talks their way to understanding.

Take notes
This is a trick that Dedeker uses with her clients all the time. It may seem silly or awkward, but taking notes is a surefire way to help you listen attentively. Not only does it help you keep track of all the twists and turns of your Spewer's speech, but it also puts a damper on the brain's tendency to start formulating a rebuttal before your partner has finished. It's best to negotiate this with your partner ahead of time—whipping out a composition book without warning in the middle of a fight isn't a good look.

Regulate your emotions and be aware of your partner's emotions
In addition to our brains coming up with all kinds of quippy responses and prying questions, our emotions can wreak havoc on our ability to listen attentively to a partner. This can be true even in relatively innocuous situations—your partner is venting about a bad interaction with their mother and it's starting to bum you out. Or your partner is bubbling over with excited energy about a new job offer in a different city, and you're already feeling anxious about how you're going to make it work. In more heated situations, such as sitting and listening to your partner spew about all the exact ways that you hurt their feelings, it gets even more challenging.

Emotional regulation doesn't mean stuffing down your feelings, pretending that they don't exist, or striving to become an enlightened being who doesn't feel anything at all. It means regularly taking a temperature check: What's going on inside? Is my heart racing? Am I breathing faster? Do I feel a rush of anger? Sadness? You know your inner workings best, and you are the best authority on which clues to watch out for. If you're noticing emotional activation that is making it difficult to listen, it's a great time to call a time-out to get what you need. That could be a twenty-minute break, a drink of water, a walk around the block, a comforting touch, or it could just be a solid clarifying question to help understand your partner's position.

IF YOUR PARTNER IS A CHEWER . . .

Agree ahead of time on a check-in ritual

Having a regular check-in like a RADAR (see Chapter 7) can do wonders for helping your resident Chewer feel safe. Knowing in advance the time, place, and topics allows space for chewing and getting thoughts in order without being under pressure. Of course, it's not always convenient or possible to save processing-heavy topics of conversation for a check-in that may be happening in weeks. We encourage the art of pausing when a discussion gets heavy and agreeing on a future time and place to revisit the topic. Even if the revisit takes place just an hour later, it still affords a clear time for your Chewer to work through their thoughts.

Keep yourself occupied without escalating

Whether you are a Chewer or a Spewer yourself, it can be challenging to hang tight and stay calm while your partner is taking personal time to process. In their absence, a vacuum is created, and there are all kinds of dreadful things waiting to fill that vacuum: pouting, ruminating, creating stories about what your partner is thinking and feeling, fixating on all the snappy comebacks you're going to throw at them when they get back, or getting so emotionally worked up that you go storming after your partner, demanding that they continue the conversation right then and there.

The best way to deal with the vacuum is to proactively choose something healthy to fill it with. At the very least, find an activity that will occupy your focus and prevent you from sitting and stewing. In the short term, this could be an engaging movie, video game, book, or hobby. In the long term, it may be helpful to rope in self-care practices that help you stay calm and regulated, such as meditating, journaling, self-touch, or whatever helps you to feel safe and secure.

Find a safe person or place to process with in the meantime

Your partner going off to chew is also a good opportunity to do some processing of your own. Regardless of your processing style, your partner going off to chew may be a welcome relief, giving you a chance to process as well. Or it may be a destabilizing shock, leaving you reeling and unsure. In addition to the activities above for keeping yourself grounded and occupied, find somewhere or someone safe enough to help you process in the way that works best for you. Write in a journal, call up a trusted friend, or connect with a therapist. Whatever you do, don't clamp down on all your thoughts and feelings and try to white knuckle it. While keeping up a stoic and controlled façade may seem to work in the short term, the drain on your mental and emotional energy is going to leave you depleted and less prepared to revisit the conversation in a healthy way.

> ## EMILY SAYS
>
> When I was in a relationship with Jase, we tended to process ideas and conflicts in similar ways. We both are Spewers, so when we talked about something that was percolating in our minds, it was common that we would not have fully formed ideas when we were in the midst of a conversation. This also made disagreements a little easier to cope with because our communication style is so similar. When I entered into a relationship with my current partner, Josh, it was almost like I had to learn a new language. Josh is such a Chewer, and he would often ask for more time to think about a conversation or a conflict that we just had. That gap in the time it took to resolve a conversation was challenging for me at first, but I have learned to really appreciate getting my own time to think and reflect while he is doing the same, quietly, in a different room. We are now able to give some space to our conflicts so that we can both come back together with less heightened emotions and a more objective understanding of the issue at hand.

Combination Station

There are a number of different combinations of processing styles that are possible in two-person relationships. Having the same processing style as a partner does not automatically guarantee success, and having a different processing style from a partner does not automatically mean it's doomed to fail. Here are some unique strengths and challenges you may be facing, depending on how you are matched up. If a particular strength or challenge seems familiar to you, it may be a clue as to which processing styles you and your partner are working with.

Chewer & Chewer

Strengths:

- May bring lots of careful deliberation to joint decision-making.

- May be better at taking pauses during conflict for both people to have time to process.

Challenges:

- Conflict could be long and drawn-out, potentially to the extent of not being fully resolved.

- Potential for both partners feeling left in the dark regarding the other person's thought process and decision-making.

Chewer & Spewer

Strengths:

- Together, you can benefit from the brainstorming powers of the Spewer to throw out possibilities and express possible emotions while having the Chewer to rein them in.

- The Chewer can provide the benefit of coming back to a discussion with more insights and information that a Spewer alone couldn't have worked through.

Challenges:

- May completely misattune, misunderstand, or miscommunicate with each other.

- One or both people may be convinced that their processing style is "correct" and seek to change their partner.

Spewer & Spewer

Strengths:

- Disagreements may be resolved quickly as both people are motivated to air their thoughts and grievances immediately.

- Both partners may feel assured that the other person is not concealing their true feelings or avoiding speaking honestly for the sake of keeping the peace.

Challenges:

- Disagreements may escalate and get off track easily as each person brings in multiple different threads.

- Discussions can become quite lengthy in order to accommodate each person being able to fully process.

EXTRA CONSIDERATIONS FOR NONMONOGA-MOUS CHEWERS AND SPEWERS

If you have multiple partners or even a closely knit circle of friends, you will have some extra experiences and interactions between different communication styles. There are a few additional things to keep in mind to help make all of those relationships feel good.

With more than two people, there are exponentially more possible combinations. If you are in a triad, quad, or other relationship where multiple people are having to communicate with each other on a regular basis, being aware of individual processing styles can still be helpful. Awareness and metacommunication are key.

Let's take a triad composed of two Chewers and one Spewer. The Spewer may feel at odds and put out by the "dominant" culture of chewing within the relationship. Or the Chewers may feel at the mercy of the Spewer and feel pressure to go along with the more vocal Spewer's decision-making. Have conversations early and often to generate understanding about each other's processing styles and come up with ideas for helping everyone get what they need.

- Keeping track of each person's processing style can take a little extra work. When you are first learning about Chewers and Spewers, you may need to do additional mental work to remember who has what style and to make adjustments to how you might communicate with them in order to make you all feel safe and appreciated.

- Avoid teaming up or making judgments about one style being better than the other. For the three of us, Emily and Jase are Spewers and Dedeker is a Chewer. It could be easy to fall into a two-against-one mind-set, trying to prove that Spewers are superior, but that doesn't help improve any of our communication.

- Having multiple simultaneous relationships can give you a power-up when it comes to identifying others' processing styles. You are able to see the differences in your partners clearly when you compare how your discussions go. This can also give you a lot of insight into your own style, by seeing how you compare to your partners in terms of how much you want to talk through something or how much you want space and time to figure it out.

Troubleshooting: No Excuses

This chapter's troubleshooting section is going to take a different format. Applying the label of "Chewer" or "Spewer" to your own processing style can be liberating. As we discussed earlier, using labels may feel constraining for some, while offering others a much-needed shorthand to quickly and efficiently describe what they need to take care of themselves. The unfortunate side effect of this is that the label can also act like a Band-Aid that covers up and excuses less than savory behavior. In the interest of living up to the *Multiamory* motto of "Don't weaponize this shit!" here are some behaviors to avoid:

Chewing is not an excuse for stonewalling.
Stonewalling is when you ignore a partner by refusing to speak, answer questions, respond to text messages, or otherwise engage with them in a meaningful way. This includes giving the silent treatment, only giving monosyllabic grunts in response, or walking out the door without saying a word. Stonewalling is included in the Gottman Institute's list of relationship-destroying behaviors, which they have called "The Four Horsemen of the Apocalypse" in relationships. What distinguishes stonewalling from chewing? Care and communication. Take care of both yourself and your partner by communicating the when, where, and how long you need to chew.

Spewing is not an excuse for steamrolling.
Everyone wants to be heard and valued. No one wants to be steamrolled. Spewing and processing externally are good, but not if they come at the expense of the other person getting a word in edgewise. This can be a problem for non-Spewers as well, particularly if you grew up in a household where interruption and steamrolling others was the only way to be heard. This is why self-awareness and self-limits are so important here. If you know that your verbal processing can be long-winded, defend your partner's right to share and be heard by being aware of the time and space that you are taking up.

Chewing is not an excuse for conflict avoidance.
As much as we advocate for taking breaks and time away as part of a chewing plan, this too can be misused. Calling for a pause in order to have chewing time can be a much-needed emergency EJECT button from a difficult conversation, but this can go haywire if it becomes a permanent break from the conflict altogether. Endlessly extending requests for chewing time can be used

as an avoidance tactic, acting as an excuse to escape the mental and emotional labor of processing your own feelings and leaving your partner in the lurch. Take the time that you need, but make sure you're actually moving toward resolution.

Spewing is not an excuse for unfiltered critique.
Spewing is like a spigot. Don't turn it on full blast. "Full blast" means throwing all filters in the garbage and letting your partner really have it with criticism, insults, personal attacks, faultfinding, or tactless observations. There are few of us who haven't thought, *You're being a real asshole* in the wake of feeling hurt by a partner. However, it's important to keep in mind that the person on the receiving end of your processing is a living, breathing human being. We recommend *compassionate* honesty rather than *radical* honesty. This is another place where finding an alternate person to spew to can come in handy. A trusted friend or a reliable therapist may be a more appropriate place to toss out all the raw feelings.

Homework

For this chapter, we recommend a journaling exercise that will help you not only understand your own processing style but also get better at recognizing and accommodating the styles of others. For each prompt below, jot down some answers in a journal, online document, or note-taking app, and come back to review whenever you need.

- What processing styles have you noticed in others around you? Think about your caregivers, your family, your best friend, your work colleagues. Have the processing styles of others around you influenced your own?

- Have you ever been punished or shamed by others for having your particular processing style? Which memories stand out for you? For Chewers, this could be raised voices from a parent for not having an answer right away. For Spewers, this might be memories of a scolding from a friend for being too talkative.

- Have you ever punished or shamed someone else for their particular processing style? Are there times in the past where you've felt frustrated or hurt by someone's processing style?

After taking some time to reflect and write down your thoughts about the prompts above, it can be helpful to get your partners, friends, or family members on board. Anyone you want to have a more intentional relationship with could benefit from reading this chapter, doing the homework prompts, and then sharing your findings together.

Sit down with your partner/friend/colleague/family member and take turns sharing what you know about your own processing style. If it's appropriate, collaborate on a spewing/chewing plan to help establish best practices for caring for each other.

Takeaways

- Some people tend to process their thoughts out loud and share each thought as it comes, while others prefer to process internally and only share once they have reached a conclusion.

- Spewers, or external processors, thrive on collaboration and brainstorming while they work things out. They need to be careful, however, to let others know that these might not be full thoughts yet and they are just speaking out loud in order to process.

- Chewers, or internal processors, crave time to work out their thoughts and feelings about something on their own before being asked to share with others. They may need to assure others that they are thinking about something and that they aren't avoiding a conversation.

- Your processing style may be enhanced by or be completely distinct from other aspects of yourself, such as your attachment style, level of introversion or extroversion, or gender identity.

- Understanding your processing style as well as others' can be incredibly powerful in improving your communication and allowing you to communicate what your own process is while respecting theirs.

For more information, check out *Multiamory* Episode 264, "Are you a Chewer or a Spewer?"

| **Microscripts:**
Secret Codes for
Communication

T ara and Juliet were in the thick of their morning routine: getting the kid dressed, whipping up breakfast smoothies, and feeding the dogs. Just as Tara was about to leave for work, she popped her head back into the kitchen, where Juliet was rinsing dishes.

"I have a late client meeting today, so I need you to take the kiddo to his doctor's appointment."

"Okay," Juliet uttered without looking up from the sink.

Tara paused, ruffled by Juliet's terseness. She took a step into the kitchen.

"I told you last night that this might be a possibility today. Is it a problem now?"

Juliet looked up, annoyed. "It's not a problem. I already said that when we talked about it last night."

"Then why did you react that way?"

"I didn't react in *any* way! All I said was 'okay'!"

"Well, you don't *sound* okay!"

This is what we like to call a "nothing fight." Nothing fights are the little quibbles and day-to-day altercations that are easy to fall into with a romantic partner, especially if you're living together. Often, the stakes are low. Neither person feels like they have much skin in the game at first. Both parties may even ultimately be in agreement. And yet, somehow, a fight kicks off before either person realizes what hit them.

Nothing fights often start with small, innocuous triggers: a sigh, a facial expression, or a particular tone of voice. That trigger gets met with a negative reaction from the other person, which starts to escalate the conversation. Memories of painful experiences from the past swoop in to color both people's perceptions, and then everyone gets sucked down a familiar yet unpleasant path of habitual communication patterns. If we were to turn the phenomena that produce nothing fights into a tidy formula, it might look like this:

$$\left(\begin{array}{c} \text{small trigger} \\ + \\ \text{reactivity} \\ + \\ \text{painful past experiences} \end{array} \right) \times \begin{array}{c} \text{habitual} \\ \text{communication} \\ \text{patterns} \end{array} = \text{nothing fight}$$

Nothing fights can be a clue that something deeper and more painful is at play, but generally the fight itself is a toxic combination of low stakes and high frustration. For many people, nothing fights arise more out of habit than out of necessity.

Ending Fights with Magic

Is there a magic word or phrase that can end any fight? In a word, no, but plenty of people have tried to claim that they've found the silver bullet. In the bonus episode for *Multiamory* Episode 288, we took a look at what the Internet had to say about ending an argument. Here are some gems:

Source: *Women's Health*
The claim: "This Magical Phrase Will End Almost Any Argument with Your Partner"
The magic phrase: "I see where you are coming from."
Our take: Not bad! Validating your partner is a good move. But this could easily go off the rails if you follow it up with an inaccurate, paraphrased assumption of where you *think* your partner is coming from. Then again, they did claim it would end *almost* any argument . . .

Source: *StarBiz*
The claim: "The Magic Word Which Can Save Any Relationship Fights [*sic*]"
The magic phrase: "I love you."
Our take: Sure, it helps to drop in reminders to your partner that you love them, even if you're angry or upset. But claiming this as a cure-all brings back too many memories of hearing something along the lines of "I love you . . . and if you really loved me, you would do X, Y, Z!"

Source: *WordfromtheBird.blog*
The claim: "The One Phrase That Ends a Fight Every Single Time"
The magic phrase: "I am not your enemy."
Our take: Sorry, little bird, but this seems like an escalation waiting to happen. It would be easy to interpret this as a passive accusation, which is fertile ground for defensiveness. "What are you talking about? I never said you were my enemy!"

Source: *Reader's Digest*
The claim: "The Four-Letter Word That Can End Any Fight—No, Not THAT Word!"
The magic phrase: "Ouch."
Our take: The thinking behind this is that you can stop a fight in its tracks by signaling to your partner that your feelings have gotten hurt. Unfortunately, when emotions are escalating, it can be a lot harder to flex that empathy muscle, and there's a chance that even the most generous of partners might not be ready to drop the entire conversation on a dime. Though that does inspire us to think of what other four-letter words might actually work if you randomly shouted them at your partner during a fight. CAKE!

None of these phrases are a total waste of time in principle, but we don't believe there are truly any one-size-fits-all magical solutions to end a fight (unless you are specifically having a magical duel, which will not be covered in this book. Again, please wait for the launch of *Multisorcery*).

However, we do believe that with creativity and collaboration, you and your partner can cultivate your very own, tailor-made, argument-ending magic. The key is to tap into the unique qualities of yourselves, your relationship, and your communication patterns.

Unique Relationships, Unique Problems, Unique Solutions

At *Multiamory*, we have had to spend many years taking research and resources focused on traditional relationships and translating them to apply to the vast spectrum of modern, less traditional relationships. We've also spent years hearing from listeners in all kinds of unique, challenging situations who feel left behind by conventional relationship wisdom. For us, two paradoxical truths about relationships have emerged:

TRUTH #1
There are fundamental best practices for healthy, functional communication that can be applied regardless of what type of relationship you're in, and regardless of how simple or complex the situation might be.

TRUTH #2
Every relationship and every situation involves unique problems, unique dynamics, and unique individuals that require unique solutions.

You can read every relationship book, visit every couple's counselor, and listen to every episode of *Multiamory*, but at the end of the day, you know your relationship the best. You are the most qualified person to design communication solutions for your unique relationship. Think of yourself as the number one professionally certified wizard called in to drum up some custom magic for the recurring arguments particular to you and your relationships.

We like to call that magic . . . Microscripts!

Microscripts: An Introduction

A Microscript is a short, predetermined interaction between you and another person, designed to interrupt old patterns and act as a shortcut to healthier communication. Microscripts have two important pieces: a cue and a script. Simply put, the *cue* is the pattern, prompt, or situation that acts as a signal for starting up the *script*, which is the word, phrase, brief dialogue, or action that follows.

First, let's talk about the cue. Old patterns and dysfunctional communication can come about as a result of assumptions you and your partner have made about one another, moments of emotional overwhelm and stress, trauma responses, habits picked up from past relationships or family of origin, and more. Some possible cues could be when you notice that you and your partner are ramping up to the same argument about the dishes that you've had about once a week for months. It could be when you're starting to fall into the usual back-and-forth about deciding what to do for dinner. Or it might be when you feel yourself tensing up right as your partner asks for a favor. Later in the chapter, we'll take a deeper dive into which situations are most appropriate for a Microscript, but the underlying principle for finding a cue is simple: whatever way you and your partner have been communicating, it's the stuff that ain't working that you wanna fix.

Once the cue is clear, then the script follows. This is the word, phrase, brief dialogue, or action that you and your partner undertake when the agreed-upon cue arises. This script should be brief and feel easy to complete. It can be hard to imagine communicating in a different way from how you've always done so up to this point, and it can be especially difficult to imagine an easy, breezy, or playful replacement. But if you and your partner can collaborate and bring your creative A-game, that script can take a tense situation and change it into a moment of laughter and love.

After realizing they were falling into patterns of nothing fights, Tara and Juliet found that creating a Microscript together was the best way to disrupt their bad habit. First, they looked for the cue. When they sat down to talk it out, they realized while neither of them ever felt excited about taking on extra chores such as taking out the trash, bringing the kid to the doctor, or troubleshooting the printer, they both agreed that these things were necessary tasks that they were willing to perform with more enthusiasm. They also both valued their family and their relationship, and they were amenable to doing extra when asked in order to help each other out.

"We're on the same page about what it takes to keep our home running in a way that keeps everyone happy," Juliet realized. "The problem is how each of us accepts that sort of request from the other. That's when our communication tends to fall apart."

Their conversation went even deeper, and Tara and Juliet uncovered some valuable insight about each other's backgrounds. Juliet grew up with a supermom who excelled at carrying the mental load for running the household. This included things like keeping track of the kids' school assignments, managing the family calendar, keeping a mental inventory of the pantry, and much more. Juliet's dad was a loving and engaged father, but he often relied on Juliet's mom to be the family expert. He would give a simple "Okay, honey" to any task requested of him. This pattern in her parents' relationship made an impression on Juliet and eventually played out in her own coparenting relationship.

Tara grew up in a family where communication often started out passive-aggressive but sometimes escalated to being *actually* aggressive. Countless times she watched her mother react to her stepfather's criticism by giving a strained "Okay" through gritted teeth. Everyone in the household knew that it wouldn't be long before an explosive fight would occur. Tara knew that she had to do whatever she could to placate her mother as quickly as possible, or else get the heck out of there. After comparing notes, it was clear to the two of them how even an innocuous word like "Okay" could produce completely different responses!

Then, it was time to decide on a script. Tara and Juliet knew they wanted a Microscript that would let them create a more positive interaction while injecting some levity into the day-to-day grind of errands. Their Microscript was simple: when one of them asked for a favor or reminded the other of a household task, they agreed to simply respond with "Ready!"—usually accompanied by a cheesy grin or a superhero pose. They both thought it was silly but decided to give it a try.

"It's pretty remarkable how much this Microscript introduced humor and laughter into our daily life!" said Tara, after she and Juliet had used the Microscript for a few weeks. "Even though the initial luster has worn off, we still keep using it because it's working." Even at times when they could barely muster the energy to say, "Ready!" it still served to signal an opportunity to perform an act of service for one another. The message behind the word "Ready!" was "I may not be excited to take on this task, but I value you and our family, so I'll do it. We both know it's not a fun task, but I'm willing to help, and you don't need to feel bad for asking me to do it." That's a lot of important meaning to load into a single word and gesture!

What You'll Need

We'll take you through a step-by-step process for creating your own Microscripts, but first, there are some important skills to cover. Think of this as the "what you'll need" or "ingredients and materials" section of a crafting project:

SELF-AWARENESS

Cultivating self-awareness can be challenging, and that pursuit is made even more difficult in romantic relationships. When in a relationship, it's easy to get emotionally charged by a partner's criticism, sarcastic facial expression, or dismissive scoff, and it's often difficult to objectively parse out how you might be contributing to cyclical problems yourself. Self-awareness means having a deep understanding of your emotional life as well as an ability to look outside yourself and assess how your actions are affecting those around you. It takes a tremendous amount of introspection and understanding of your personal history, your cognitive biases, and your limitations to be able to evaluate your part in habitual communication breakdowns.

Most of us don't do this. It would be easier to blame our partners for all our collective relationship problems, right? And in certain relationships, abuse, coercion, and gaslighting are all justifiable reasons to seek help or leave. But in partnerships where "nothing fights" and communication breakdowns are prevalent, cultivating self-awareness can enact an enormous positive change. So, the next time you find yourself getting in yet another fight with your partner over who does the dishes, ask yourself, how am I contributing to the argument? What are my personal hang-ups regarding this issue? When and why do I find myself having strong emotional reactions over seemingly minor things? Pursuing self-awareness and an ability to step back and look at the bigger picture is our first prerequisite when beginning the work of breaking bad habitual patterns and creating Microscripts with your partner.

A WILLINGNESS TO METACOMMUNICATE
We previously talked about the importance of metacommunication in Chapter 2. As a refresher, metacommunication refers to the ability to communicate about how you communicate. It is crucial that there are channels open for you or your partner to

call out or reflect on patterns that aren't working in a way that feels safe and productive.

It's important to remember that your family of origin, your personal history, and the unique styles in which you communicate (check out Chapter 3 for more information on communication styles) all contribute to how you view the world around you and how your communication lands on your partner. Most likely your partner will not have the same experiences as you, and therefore the way they view the world and their communication style may be vastly different from yours. Being able to share vulnerably and communicate effectively with one another about these things is a key step in creating effective Microscripts.

A TEAM MENTALITY

We've all been in situations where we feel like we're at odds with our partner. It's us vs. them, and we are in a cage match to determine the winner. We throw insults, spout criticisms, and roll our eyes to let them know just how much we are hurt by something that they have said or done. After all, if we don't like something that our partner did, shouldn't they just stop doing it? Sometimes the answer is yes. Maybe in some scenarios your partner isn't acting appropriately, and perhaps they should work toward changing a specific behavior. Often, however, arguments with our partners are more nuanced than figuring out who's right and who's wrong, and solutions are not always black or white.

Ideally when we are beginning to craft Microscripts with a partner, we will work to shift our focus away from a "you vs. me" mentality and move toward an "us vs. the problem" mentality. This is a crucial change in mind-set and can be a necessary shift to help your relationship thrive. A "you vs. me" mentality can be devastating to your relationships on many levels, as well as your outlook on how you operate and exist in the world. An article by Arash Emamzadeh in *Psychology Today* describes this type of mentality on a more global level as "oversimplifying and distorting complex problems by dividing the world into an us and a them, and scapegoating and vilifying the latter." While this definition may sound alarmist when applied to relationships, this type of mentality over long periods of time can wreak havoc on your romantic life. It can breed resentment, distrust, and anxiety and lead to an irreconcilable fracturing of the relationship. Remember that you and your partner are on the same team. A Microscript doesn't exist for the purpose of getting just one person to shape up their communication—instead it exists for both of you to collaborate in reconciling a problem.

ABILITY TO SELF-SOOTHE

Being able to drop a code word with a silly grin is all fine and good, but what about the moments when you are really, *really* annoyed with your partner? Even when special care and time are taken to create a Microscript, there is still the potential for negative habitual emotions to rear their ugly heads when tension is brewing. A key to keeping your cool in many challenging situations lies in accessing the ability to self-soothe when you most need it. Self-soothing can help bring you back into the moment, calm your nervous system, and remind your psyche that you are safe and cared for. Self-soothing tactics can be as simple as taking three deep breaths when you feel anxiety or anger rising to the surface. It could mean removing yourself from the situation by doing things like exiting the room, taking a walk around the block, meditating for ten minutes, or breaking out into a mini yoga session! With practice, whipping out your Microscript at the appropriate moment will become second nature.

HOW TO CREATE A MICROSCRIPT

You might be reading this chapter and saying to yourself, "That's all well and good—thanks for the information—but how the heck do I actually create one of these things?" Well, you came to the right place! Here's how to create your Microscript in four simple steps, including an example of how we came up with one of our own personal Microscripts.

1. **Identify the problem:** Think about the last time you and your partner got into a fight over something. Was it a recurring fight? How did it make the two of you feel? Would you identify it as a misunderstanding, a difference in opinion, or a reluctance to perform a task? If the situation came up again, how would you two prefer the scenario play out? Discuss with your partner how you both feel when your nothing fight or tense moment occurs and how you would *like* to feel in these situations instead.

   As an example, the three of us would get distracted by our phones during long meetings or on extended recording days for *Multiamory*. Usually, one person would be the culprit and the other two would get annoyed that they weren't focusing on the task at hand. When called out on it, the person using their phone would get defensive or frustrated that someone else had used their phone earlier. This problem persisted over the course of the first few years that we were working together. After many crabby moments, we finally set aside intentional time to talk about the fact that the three of us had a pattern of letting outside forces like our phones or other work get in the way of our *Multiamory* time. We all agreed that we wanted to be focused and give our full attention to taking care of our podcast baby and that no one enjoyed having to scold someone else for being on their phone.

2. **Find the cue:** As you and your partner explore what's underneath this recurring issue, it may become clear what the catalyst is: a look, a sigh, a tone of voice, or a particular word. Or it may be less clear which domino piece is the culprit, and you may have to experiment with which cue to choose. Collaborate with your partner to pick a clear cue to work with. It's important to remember to do this *without blame, criticism, or shame*. These dysfunctional patterns are often cocreated, meaning it's not just one person's fault. That's why it's also important to cocreate a new pattern together.

   Initially, there wasn't a clear verbal cue for *Multiamory's* phone problem. However, it was obvious when someone was getting a glazed-over look or giving monosyllabic responses as they doomscrolled Twitter. We decided on a cue that happened early in the pattern. We wanted to nip distraction in the bud before it even became an issue. Instead of waiting for someone to begin to check out, we decided that the official beginning of a meeting would act as the cue.

3. **Write the script:** Now comes the fun part—time to create the Microscript! Examine the speech patterns or inside jokes that the two of you share. Can any of those be morphed into a Microscript? Get creative! Find something fun and personal that is simple and unique to your relationship.

   After realizing we needed to work on being more focused around meeting time, we created a script that was unique to our collective senses of humor, which would remind us to be focused. We decided that when we have a meeting or recording time, the first thing we do is triumphantly announce, "Phones in the garbage!" We aren't actually putting our phones in the garbage, but it acts as a signal to put them completely out of sight and to turn our attention to our work. This Microscript has had a tremendously positive effect; it's increased our productivity and shortened the length of our meetings! When someone starts to zone out, one of us will usually whip out the Microscript. However, using the Microscript at the top of our meetings has been effective enough that we rarely need it otherwise.

4. **Repeat, repeat, repeat:** Our brains are stubborn, and it takes a long time to change a habit or learn a new skill. One of the easiest ways to alter your thinking around a persistent problem is to practice using your Microscript over and over again. Remember that the Microscript helps you and your partner show that you care about one another and that you are willing to work collaboratively to fix a problem. As you try it out and use it in real life, it's also okay to make adjustments and changes to find what's best. The perfect Microscript for you is the one that works, so keep making modifications until it feels good.

   One suggestion we have for trying out a new Microscript is to make a plan together to use it for a set amount of time, and then check in to see if it's working the way you intended. If it's a script you use every day, you could practice using it for a week or two and then assess how well it is working. If it's a Microscript that doesn't need to be used as often, take it for a longer test drive of a month or more. By creating a specific time frame to practice, you free yourselves from needing to iron out the perfect Microscript immediately and instead can jump right into using it and reaping the benefits while you continue to improve it.

   Soon the Microscript will become second nature, and the issue that caused its creation may end up feeling like a thing of the past. "Phones in the garbage" is something that we still say occasionally, but the ritual of being fully present with one another during meetings is something that the three of us do automatically now.

How Microscripts Work

Microscripts aren't magical due to wishful thinking. Here's what's going on under the hood that makes Microscripts so effective:

MICROSCRIPTS INCORPORATE IDIOSYNCRATIC LANGUAGE (A.K.A. MORE IN-JOKES = BETTER RELATIONSHIPS)

One of the best parts of being in a relationship is the opportunity to create your own language with your partner. That language often consists of inside jokes or unique speech patterns that mean something important and fundamental to only the two (or three or more) of you. This language is not only created with words and phrases but may also include gestures, vocal tonality, facial expressions, terms of endearment, and more. A Microscript takes this personal, private language a step further and turns a joke or a phrase into an expression with a purpose. If a friend or family member were a fly on the wall bearing witness to the two of you using your Microscript, they might have no idea how significant that moment is. That's what's so great about Microscripts!

Microscripts work by harnessing the power of *idiosyncratic language*. That's a fancy science term for the in-jokes, code words, nicknames, and weird slang that make up the unique dialect of your personal relationships. Idiosyncratic language shows up in romantic connections, friendships, work relationships, and within families. (It also shows up among podcast hosts. Emily started calling Dedeker "DooDoo" one day during a *Multiamory* meeting, and despite initial resistance, the nickname has stuck.)

Dr. Catherine Morelock, who has been studying idiosyncratic

language for years, made an interesting discovery when she was looking at a list of phrases that couples had requested as engravings on their wedding bands. (We assume this was for research purposes, unless Dr. Morelock moonlights as a bespoke ring engraver.) There were over two hundred phrases, most of which were what you'd expect: the couple's initials, an anniversary date, or common romantic idioms like "Eternally Yours" or "Happily Ever After." But about a quarter of the phrases broke the pattern and included unusual turns of phrase, nonsensical language, or odd pet names. For these people, the unique language of their relationship was so meaningful that they had to include it on a symbol as important as their wedding ring!

Dr. Morelock's research shows that idiosyncratic language isn't just a by-product of close relationships but may actually serve to create that feeling of closeness in the first place. Dr. Morelock and other researchers have found that more frequent usage of idiosyncratic language in relationships was significantly related to feelings of closeness, fondness, and connection, as well as a sense of being truly known by one's partner.

This may be obvious at first blush. Many people get joy out of making their best friend crack up with an in-joke and feel those warm fuzzies of affection when a partner uses their favorite pet name (amazingly, even being called "DooDoo" has a positive association for Dedeker now). But what does this have to do with fights and arguments?

It turns out that idiosyncratic language is extremely powerful when used as part of a "repair attempt" during conflict. In research terms, a "repair attempt" is anything that helps to de-escalate negativity and negative feelings during a fight. This can include a variety of different behaviors, including apologies, asking to slow down, expressing appreciation, or using kind humor. Idiosyncratic communication in the form of a creative Microscript can effectively and efficiently serve any of those purposes, helping you and your partner to de-escalate an argument and tap back into feelings of kindness and positivity. You can find much more on repair attempts in the Extra Tools section.

This may be easier said than done. Whipping out a cheesy Microscript during conflict requires flexibility, trust, and the willingness to risk "losing" the argument in that moment. It takes guts to make that emotional shift from being on the defensive to actively reminding yourself and your partner that you are still dorky best friends who refer to your personal triggers as "pokies."

Meredith Bombar and Lawrence Littig Jr., researchers who studied the use of idiosyncratic baby talk in adult relationships, summed it up well:

"The abandonment of 'normal' adult roles—namely, being assertive in requesting that one's own needs be met while simultaneously being willingly vulnerable, nurturant, endearing, and silly—may prove to be more facilitating, or even necessary, for intimate personal connection than many people think."

MICROSCRIPTS CAN REWIRE YOUR BRAIN

It is easy to get caught in old communication patterns, especially in long-term relationships. Set-in patterns that you inherited from your family of origin or past relationships can start to run the show, causing communication breakdowns as small as day-to-day nothing fights or as large as relationship-ending blowouts. The good news is that these communication patterns are not a death sentence, thanks to the power of neuroplasticity.

Neuroplasticity is the brain's ability to form new synapses and reorganize neural pathways in response to the environment. Everything from learning a new skill to going through a period of extreme stress can functionally rewire your brain, for better or worse. Neuroplastic activity is at its highest during childhood, when literally everything around you is a learning experience that your brain is adapting to. A growing body of evidence suggests that our brains retain their plasticity throughout life, enabling us to adapt to changing life circumstances.

This means that it is possible to turn around habitual reactions and communication even though the neural pathways may run deep. Microscripts serve as a sort of circuit breaker that not only interrupts the pattern but provides a new pattern to follow, laying the groundwork for your brain to create a new connection around whatever used to set off the old pattern. Over time, the new neural pathway grows more robust and reliable, becoming second nature. We think it's much better to collaborate with your partner on a Microscript that proactively encourages your brain and communication to fire in the direction that you want it to go, rather than just leaving it up to chance.

JASE SAYS

It is easy for me to fall into particular negative thought patterns and reactions. I have a repertoire of some of my favorite moves, such as blaming myself for anything that goes wrong, negating any compliments I receive, taking random statements personally, being quick to react to a perceived insult, and many more. Discovering Microscripts and having a partner who also values them has been a game changer for me.

When it comes to rejecting compliments, Dedeker is a champion at reminding me of my Microscripts and saying something like, "You're right!" when I receive a compliment rather than deflecting or arguing with it. I think the biggest impact for us, though, has been in disrupting that classic

---

pattern where resentment builds over a particular habit or idiosyncrasy and causes pointless arguments or fights. We've gotten good at identifying that building tension early (usually at a RADAR) and then brainstorming Microscripts to try. They usually involve rhymes or jokes that are so inside that it would take an entire chapter to explain (and you would probably be rolling your eyes the whole time). For us, the more tongue-in-cheek or ridiculously nonsensical, the better. "Live. Laugh. Lokes." has saved the day countless times by turning frustration into humor and connection (and no, I'm not going to try to explain that one).

MICROSCRIPTS LET YOU TAKE A BREATH

There's nothing worse than finding yourself in the throes of a fight that turned nasty after a small communication misunderstanding or a poorly worded comment. In those moments, it's easy to get caught up in heightened emotions and continue to say things you don't really mean. That's why whipping out your trusty Microscript can be so important before things escalate and the two of you get dragged into the weeds. Your Microscript can offer a chance for stabilization in a tense moment. Ideally, if you find yourself in a situation where anger or resentment is bubbling to the surface, choose to take a breath and whip out your Microscript! It can turn an emotionally charged event on its head and invite in laughter and understanding. We can't choose our emotional life, but we can choose what actions we are going to take at any given moment. A Microscript is a codified tool to help you communicate with your partner, push past your initial reaction, and transcend the unreliability of your heightened emotions.

MICROSCRIPTS DEPERSONALIZE THE PROBLEM

As humans, we are fantastic at getting caught up in our own stories regarding any issue in communication. This often means that we project our problems onto others, take things super personally, and fail to cut our partners slack when they most need it. And, if these patterns become habits, they can truly wreak havoc on the overall health of a relationship. That's why it is so important to create tools that allow the two of you to separate a problem from the individual. Eri Kardos, relationship coach and author of *Relationship Agreements*, has a distinct take on this. "There are actually three unique entities in any one partnership. You + Them + The Relationship. You can care for your relationship as a separate entity by making space for all three."

In our interview with Kardos in *Multiamory* Episode 103, she gave the example of calling a relationship "Fred" and visualizing Fred as a cute, furry blue monster. The people in the relationship have to care for Fred and nurture it as it grows and evolves. Whether you view your relationship as a blue monster, a unicorn, or a bright beam of light, we love the idea of separating yourselves from the relationship itself. With a Microscript, the problem also becomes separate, and the two of you are simply nurturing the relationship by creating a tool that is helping depersonalize and tackle the specific issue. In the care and feeding of your relationship, there is nothing too zany or off-the-wall if it resonates for the two of you.

MICROSCRIPTS CAN SERVE AS AN IMPORTANT RITUAL

Some relationship rituals can be toxic. Does this one sound familiar? Every time your partner lets the door or kitchen cabinet slam shut, you grimace and snidely remind them how loud they are being. They roll their eyes and tell you they'll be quieter. You chuckle to yourself and say, "That's what you said last time." A fight ensues, and a week later the same thing happens. Lather, rinse, repeat. The ritual of nothing fights such as this can take a tremendous toll on a relationship over a long period of time.

However, there is research indicating that *positive* rituals can increase relationship satisfaction and aid in relationship quality and longevity. Our Microscripts can, in essence, become positive rituals to replace the negative patterns that we once got sucked into. These rituals might not come easily to you at first. We love to apply the "fake it till you make it" affirmation to our Microscripts in early use. Eventually, the Microscript will become rote and might even morph into something sillier or quirkier as your relationship deepens. But until then, practice makes perfect! Smile, Microscript, repeat.

You Might Need a Microscript If . . .

We don't recommend using Microscripts for every single relationship predicament, but here's a handy list of situations where we've seen Microscripts being particularly effective, complete with examples:

YOU NOTICE YOURSELF THINKING, "MY PARTNER *ALWAYS* REACTS LIKE _____." OR "MY PARTNER *NEVER* DOES _____."

Many relationship resources warn people against using the terms *always* and *never* when talking to a partner, especially when describing their behavior. These words are absolute enough that they can easily set the other person on the defensive, starting any conflict off on the wrong foot. But, if you find yourself *thinking* those words in the first place, that can be an important insight. This could be a clue about ongoing patterns that aren't working. And Microscripts are all about changing patterns!

First, it's important to bring some curiosity and questioning:

- Is this observation true?

- Can I think of any examples to the contrary where my partner behaved differently?

- What kind of response or behavior from my partner am I longing for in this situation?

- What kind of response or behavior could I have in order to set my partner up for success in this situation?

Your answers to these questions introduce even more clues about what communication patterns are taking place and what might be an effective Microscript to interrupt that pattern. After you've done some inquiry, have a conversation with your partner (ideally at a time when you're both calm and collected), and collaborate on a Microscript together.

Example: Sad Piano
Morgan came home from a long shift at work, and their partner, Alex, asked them how their day went. Morgan sighed, shrugged their shoulders, and in a defeated voice said, "Fine." Alex could tell Morgan wasn't really fine but figured they just didn't want to talk about it. In Alex's family while growing up, if you prodded someone to open up, they would get angry and insist they were okay before storming out of the room. Morgan, however, grew up in an emotional household, and to them a sigh and shrug were clear signs that they wanted someone to comfort and ask them what was wrong. Because of this, Morgan would get upset with Alex, thinking that she just didn't care about how they were feeling, and Alex would become angry that she had been misled about what Morgan needed.

After this cycle happened a few times, Morgan and Alex got into an argument. "You never care how I'm doing and just ignore me when I've had a hard day or if I'm upset about something!"

"I'm always here for you! You're the one who never opens up to me. Instead, you always end up sulking when I can't read your mind!" replied Alex, flabbergasted at the accusation.

Luckily for Morgan and Alex, they had enough metacommunication skills that after they had both calmed down, they were able to come together and brainstorm solutions. They had listened to our episode about Microscripts and realized that this could be a perfect opportunity to create one. They were consistently using "always" and "never" language in regard to this problem, and both of them struggled to reconcile their different upbringings.

In their brainstorming, they decided to make a Microscript that could work for either person, whether Alex required clarification about Morgan's state of being or Morgan wanted to make it clearer that they needed care and attention. The two decided if Morgan felt hurt that Alex wasn't asking questions when Morgan was clearly having a bad day, instead of assuming that Alex was intentionally avoiding connection, Morgan would hang their head and hum the sad Charlie Brown song "Christmas Time Is Here," as parodied on the show *Arrested Development*. This would prompt Alex to spring into action, ready to offer comfort and ask about their day, by exclaiming, "The doctor is in!"

From the other side, if Morgan seemed like they might be upset, but Alex wasn't sure if they wanted to discuss it, Alex could say, "Is that a piano playing?" and Morgan could either respond by singing the sad Charlie Brown song or just say, "No, I don't hear any piano" if they didn't need support. While all this may seem silly, having set phrases that don't include the direct question of "Do you want to talk about it?" makes inquiry easier to respond to when emotions are heightened. The silliness of the interaction also helped act as a circuit breaker and prevented them from falling back into their old patterns. The sheer nonsensicalness of the interaction injected just enough humor that it stopped them from going down their well-worn paths, reinforced the idea that they were a team, and showed them that they had a unique, special bond with one another.

You feel too overwhelmed by feelings to respond in a healthy way.

When emotions run high and conversation is tense, our ability to respond in a measured, mature, and gentle way is often the first thing to go out the window. Once that's gone, often what's left are bad habits, emotional upheaval, and trauma responses, which are more than happy to take the wheel and drive the interaction into the ground. A short, agreed-upon Microscript can be the key to stopping a negative spiral in its tracks.

In these situations, it's important to keep your Microscripts *micro*. In the heat of intense emotion, it may be too difficult to access therapist-approved wording like, "I am experiencing a lot of challenging emotions, which is making it difficult for me to listen. I would like to take a short break to regulate myself before coming back to this conversation." When you feel like you're ready to burst at the seams and your hair is going to spontaneously combust, whipping out something as simple as, "Freeze-frame!" may be a lot easier to both remember and say out loud.

Example: Thank you for your honesty

When it comes to fostering healthy, honest communication with someone, it's easy to imagine a world where you are both perfectly frank when sharing and perfectly reasonable when receiving. In reality, however, it can be downright challenging or even feel impossible to keep our cool when our partner tells us something that upsets us, even if we asked them for the information in the first place. If we react by flying off the handle each time this happens, we end up creating a situation where being honest with us doesn't feel safe. As a result, our partners might reasonably try to be a little less frank and a little more "tactful," which goes against our goals of honest and clear communication.

So what can we do about it? You guessed it: Microscripts! This example comes from the amazing blog *Polyammering* by Phoebe Philips. In her post "The Honesty Exchange," she tackles this very problem of trying to create a relationship where your partner feels safe to be honest with you, even when you might still struggle to hear that honesty. It's written in the context of a polyamorous partner talking about their date with another partner, but the principle applies to any area where hearing the truth can be difficult and require some processing. Here is her Microscript:

> *"I have a very simple default response when I'm being told a truth that I don't enjoy hearing . . . When someone gives you information that you know to be true, but that is causing you some emotional distress—the default response is to say the following: 'Thank you for your honesty.'"*

In this article, Phi is focusing on finding a way to receive difficult information tactfully and to buy herself time to process it. As a Microscript that is understood by both parties, it takes on an extra power. If you know that the phrase *Thank you for your honesty* is a Microscript for processing difficult information, it can serve as a cue that your partner appreciates your courage to share, that they acknowledge you, *and* that they need some time to process the information. This lets you know to give them a little time to process, not because you did something wrong, but because that's their own personal need.

NEURODIVERSITY AND PTSD

Not everyone's communication is the same. We all come from different backgrounds and different past experiences, and we also have brains that function in different ways. There is a whole beautiful spectrum of neurodiversity, everything from fundamental differences in brain function to temporary mental health difficulties. Your individual brain makeup can provide unique strengths as well as unique challenges, especially if you're with a partner whose brain functions differently than yours.

Dedeker shares how a good Microscript really helped her through a period of intense mental health struggles from PTSD:

After leaving a physically abusive relationship, it took a few months for PTSD symptoms to start manifesting. I found myself completely thrown off and confused by my brain and body as I experienced both physical and emotional upheaval on a daily basis. Sometimes the triggers were obvious, and sometimes they seemed to be random and obscure. It was starting to have an effect on my relationships, and my partners were at just as much of a loss as I was. Getting into therapy helped me start my healing process, as well as giving me more tools and understanding for what was going on. As part of that process, Jase and I came up with our "puffer fish" Microscript.

One day when I felt a wave of triggery symptoms coming on, I described them to Jase as being like a puffer fish. A short while later, that inspired this simple Microscript:

Dedeker: I'm feeling like a puffer fish right now.

Jase: Okay! Do you want some space, or should I put on my fish gloves?

Dedeker: Put on the fish gloves, please.

This nonsensical conversation wouldn't make sense to anyone not in the know, and it even felt silly to say the script aloud. However, it was absolutely key in my ability to care for myself by being honest about what was going on in my brain while still being connected and communicative with my partner. Having the short puffer fish phrase to lean on meant that I didn't have to go into deep detail about flashbacks or memories that were coming up, which meant that I could convey what was going on without risking the trigger getting even worse. Jase was able to give me a choice about what I needed, and I was able to pick what would be best for me in the moment without having to think about it too hard.

In case you're wondering, "fish gloves" meant that Jase would put on the metaphorical equivalent of those chain-mail gloves that people in shark cages wear in order to lovingly feed chum to a shark without losing multiple fingers. For him it meant being emotionally available, gentle, and comforting without taking my PTSD prickliness too personally.

The topic feels so awkward, you're not sure what to say.

Even the most skillful communicators run into topics where good old-fashioned discomfort and awkwardness can make it hard to communicate effectively. You may be extremely comfortable talking about sex but find that the topic of money makes you clam up. Your partner may happily overshare when it comes to talking about their childhood but struggle to know how to discuss what's going on in their other relationships. It happens to the best of us.

Unfortunately, shame, awkwardness, and embarrassment can

sabotage good communication. At best, you may find yourself stumbling over your words while feeling like your face is about to burst into flames. At worst, you may resort to changing the subject, keeping secrets, making omissions, or using other questionable behavior in order to avoid a topic altogether.

Microscripts can come to the rescue when there's an awkward topic that you're not sure how to broach. By being short and sweet and maybe even a little silly, you can defuse tension and start generating more comfort and ease with practice.

Sex is often an awkward topic, even in progressive, sex-positive relationships, but it serves as a great opportunity for you and your partner to collaborate on Microscripts and create some communication rituals. Initiating sex, accepting a sexual invitation, negotiating play, and turning down sex are all ripe for creating some agreed-upon Microscripts to help ease the conversation.

Example: Naked Time!
Darren and Grace both enjoyed their sexual connection. They had good chemistry, but as so often happens, life would get in the way, resulting in their desires not always lining up. Both of them worked demanding day jobs, and each had side projects or contract work on top of that, and it was getting harder and harder to get in a romantic mood when they were together. There had been a few times when one of them had tried to initiate sexy time with some kissing, but the other was still in "work brain" or just plain exhausted, which led to the uncomfortable process of one person having to shut down those advances. This left both of them feeling disappointed, and they struggled to come up with a less awkward way to initiate physical intimacy.

They had both learned that even if they weren't quite in the mood when they started getting intimate, usually their bodies would quickly begin to get aroused, and they would both end up having a great time. So the challenge was mostly in getting started. They found that one of the best ways was to simply lie naked together in bed. They would begin to cuddle, and that skin-to-skin contact would usually lead to sex. Even if they ended up too tired to follow all the way through, it was nice to have some physical touch for a little while. There were still times, however, when one of them was so mentally preoccupied that they didn't want to engage in any intimacy, so they decided to add a Microscript into the mix.

They set out to counter the potential disappointment of being rejected by creating an extra-silly Microscript. They had both watched a YouTube video called *Potter Puppet Pals*, which was a ridiculous parody of Harry Potter as puppets. In that video, Puppet Dumbledore would periodically show up and say, "Naked time!" It was just absurd enough that it made them laugh every time they said it, so they chose, "Would you like some naked time?" or some variation on that theme as their script. In the event that one of them just couldn't get into naked time emotionally, they could gently respond with another reference to the videos and say, "Expelliarmus!" or "I'm feeling more Avada Kedavra today." The pure absurdity of the exchange would make them smile and would take the edge off a potentially awkward and disappointing interaction.

Additional Microscript Examples

Just in case you needed additional inspiration, we've included a few more of our favorite examples from our own lives and Microscripts that have been shared with us by listeners and clients.

"I'm Full"

Microscripts don't always need to solve a serious problem with heavy emotions—they can also be used to simply make regular interactions easier and clearer. We host monthly discussion groups with podcast listeners where participants share their experiences and ask for advice or discussion from the group. Sometimes the discussion is upsetting and emotional for the person sharing, while other times it is celebratory or neutral. Regardless of the tone, we realized the person sharing sometimes needs an easy way to tell the group that it's okay to move on to talk about something else—either because they have enough to process emotionally or because they've finished discussing what they needed help with. In those cases, we came up with the Microscript saying "I'm full" when someone feels like they are satisfied with the amount of discussion on their topic.

The beauty of the "I'm full" Microscript is that it solves a number of different, small problems. For one, it takes away the stress of trying to figure out how to communicate that you are done discussing, while also removing the need to give a reason. If someone shares something vulnerable and is starting to feel over-whelmed by the discussion, they don't have to figure out a way to express that sentiment, they can simply say, "Thank you, I'm feeling full now." Similarly, if someone shares something fun and silly but they want to be respectful of other people's time and allow others to bring up topics, they also can just say, "Thanks, everyone. I'm full."

In this case, the shorthand of the Microscript allows us to more easily ask someone if they feel the topic has been discussed long enough, or if there is anything specific they are still hoping to get before moving on. This Microscript is an example of a set phrase that is used in a metaphorical way to express a variety of feelings that everyone in the discussion group can easily understand.

"Why, Thank You"

This next example is actually a combination of stories from several couples who all came up with a similar Microscript to solve a common problem. In this case, the purpose wasn't to resolve a recurring fight, but to address a negative internal habit in order to help them thrive.

Priya and Carl both had an issue that had shown up in previous relationships, with their friends, and even in their work lives: they were bad at receiving praise or taking compliments. Specifically, their default way of responding to someone saying something nice about them was to immediately deny it and explain to the person how they were wrong. This is a seriously common bad habit that all of us on the podcast occasionally fall into. In fact, in many cultures or microcultures, denial is considered the most appropriate response to kind words. The trouble is that while it may seem natural or polite, it can also make it difficult to build trust and long-term commitment if we're constantly telling ourselves and our partners that all the things they like about us are wrong or untrue. This is exactly what Carl and Priya started to notice. Not only were they telling themselves and each other that they weren't worthy of the love and affection they received, but they also both found it frustrating when they would try to give a nice, heartfelt compliment that their partner would negate! Instead of a pleasant interaction involving displays of affection, the other person would immediately tell them why they were wrong (which feels bad even if it's coming from a reaction of politeness).

Once they identified this as a problem, they started to brainstorm ways to address it. The simple answer was to say "thanks" and take the compliment. The challenge, though, was that years and years of social conditioning mixed with a large dose of internalized shame made it more difficult than they initially envisioned. When they tried to just say, "thanks," it would work for a little bit, but eventually they would fall back into their old habits.

That's the point where they embraced just a touch of silliness and created a Microscript. They decided to keep this one simple and came up with the set phrase *Why, thank you!* as a response to compliments. Something about using the old-timey phrasing made it easier for them to take the compliment and helped the other person to recognize when it was being used. Even when one of them would begin to deny a compliment by disagreeing, they had the opportunity to catch themselves and say, "Oh! I mean, why, thank you!" When they used those particular words, it was also a cue to the other person that they were working on accepting praise and trusting the fact that their partner truly meant the affection they were giving.

Another side benefit Priya discovered was that by using this Microscript, she actually began to get better at receiving compliments in general, simply by giving herself an accessible way to practice. At work or with friends, she was able to use their secret phrase, which made her smile, and nobody else had to know about it for it to work well for her.

PERSONALIZING

From the couples we've known who have decided to use similar Microscripts to the one above, we've seen some variations that either add more fun or slightly change the feeling of the Microscript to suit the couple's personalities and needs.

For one couple, they found that denying a compliment felt hurtful to the other person because it made them feel like they didn't believe their words or that they thought the other person's opinion of them was wrong. This couple decided on the phrase *You're right* to use as their Microscript. To them, it not only aided in the reception of the praise they were being given, but it also felt good to hear their partner tell them they were right about something!

Jase and Dedeker also use this Microscript when having text conversations, especially when long-distance from each other. At times when it's especially difficult to receive a compliment, they are able to simultaneously be gracious and accept the appreciation (while honestly conveying that they are struggling to do so) by typing out the phrase as "whythankyou."

Microscripts are a fun place to get creative with your partners, experiment and try out ideas, and allow them to evolve and develop over time so that they become part of your special secret language.

"Puppy Dog"

Lily and Amy were aware of the many differences in their communication, like the fact that Amy was a Spewer and Lily was a Chewer, but they made effective use of tools like the Triforce of Communication in order to metacommunicate with each other. Because they were utilizing all these tools, they were surprised to find there was a particular situation that would challenge both of them. It would happen any time they were talking about a new idea, a new trip, or a project, something that excited them both. They would be having a fun discussion when Amy would start asking all sorts of logistical questions, almost rapid-fire going through different considerations. "What would we do in this situation?" "Oh, gosh, I'll probably need to make some extra time for this. Maybe if I get up a little earlier on Fridays." "Oh, wow, this is going to be a lot to keep track of!"

As Amy continued brainstorming and asking questions, Lily

would begin to back away from the topic and get upset, because she believed the topic was stressing Amy out. Amy, however, was still keyed up, and when Lily started to withdraw, she felt hurt that Lily wasn't joining her in the excitement. After this happened a number of times, they began to notice the pattern and decided to talk it through, to understand what lines were getting crossed in this situation. In discussing it, they learned that Amy's way of expressing excitement was to ask numerous questions and to think through different angles. For her, that was part of the fun rather than being a sign of stress. From Lily's side, she had worried that Amy was getting overwhelmed and would try to shut down the conversation as a way of protecting her and avoiding that stress.

Once they identified the core difference, they decided that a Microscript could be something fun to try since they tend to be a little silly and would be a great way to add levity to the situation. In trying to describe her own state of being, Amy used the metaphor of a puppy getting excited about a walk, or playtime, or dinner, or . . . basically anything that caused it to work itself up into a frenzy that could seem stressful to someone else. This was the impetus for their Microscript. If Amy realized she was going into a hyperactive mode and felt Lily start to withdraw, she would say, "woof woof!" as a cue that she was excited and not stressed. On the other hand, if Lily saw this happening and wanted reassurance that this was a positive and not a stressful reaction, she could ask Amy if she's being a puppy dog, giving them an easy but silly way to remind themselves about their different reactions to excitement.

Homework

Microscripts can take a little practice and a great deal of trust and goodwill between you and your partner (or partners). Initially we recommend tackling something fairly innocuous that could benefit from a Microscript. You could either take one of our examples above, like "Ready" or "Why, thank you," or you could pick another area of your communication that could use a little pick-me-up and go through the four steps outlined earlier in the chapter for creating a Microscript. To recap, they are:

1. **Identify the problem:** Talk about the feelings and communication patterns you and your partner want to change. Discuss the ways you'd like to feel and communicate instead.

2. **Find the cue:** Identify a cue, such as a word, phrase, situation, or feeling that will prompt you to use the Microscript.

3. **Write the script:** Throw out some ideas of different phrases, actions, and responses that will help alleviate tension or frustration. Don't be afraid to pick some silly ones. Bonus points if it involves inside jokes or other idiosyncratic language!

4. **Repeat, repeat, repeat:** Keep using the Microscript while adjusting and refining it until it becomes second nature.

After creating a Microscript, use it for two weeks to a month and then check in with your partner on how well it is working. If you feel like it's stagnating or not giving you the results you want, go back through the steps and create a new Microscript for next month. If you still love it, continue to practice using it with one another. Create new Microscripts whenever additional conflicts arise.

Takeaways

- Every relationship and every situation involves unique problems, unique dynamics, and unique individuals that require unique solutions. Enter Microscripts!

- A Microscript is a short, predetermined interaction between you and another person designed to interrupt old patterns and act as a shortcut to healthier communication.

- Microscripts have two important parts: a cue and a script. The cue is the pattern, prompt, or situation that acts as a signal for starting up the script, which is the word, phrase, brief dialogue, or action that follows.

- You'll need to call on your self-awareness, meta-communication skills, a team mentality, and your ability to self-soothe in order to use Microscripts effectively.

- To create a Microscript, take some time with your partner to identify the problem, brainstorm what kind of replacement communication you'd rather have, decide together on a Microscript to experiment with, and then see what happens! You can always adjust it depending on how it feels.

For more information, check out *Multiamory* Episode 168, "Communication Hacks: Booster Pack."

| CHAPTER 5 | **Boundaries:** Communicate Clearly Where You Stand |

F rank and Grant were getting excited for their upcoming wedding in the fall. It had been postponed for a year due to the pandemic, and finally it was safe enough to exchange vows in front of their closest friends and family members. Frank's parents, however, were insisting that the duo invite Frank's great-aunt—a woman who was overtly homophobic.

Frank's parents were prominent lawyers and had always been incredibly generous toward Frank and his brothers. While the family was close, his parents often insisted they knew what was best, and Frank rarely stood up to their suggestions, even if he didn't agree with them. Their influence extended to many areas of his life, deciding his extracurricular activities, which Ivy League school he would attend, and which firm he would join after graduating from law school. Frank's parents loved Grant and were happy the two were finally getting married. However, since they were paying for the wedding, Frank's parents had many people they expected to be included on the guest list—including Frank's homophobic great-aunt.

Frank, ever the people pleaser, didn't want to disappoint his parents, but he knew both he and Grant had boundaries around engaging with people with homophobic attitudes. He pleaded with his parents to understand, but they kept telling him it would be fine and that they didn't want to hurt her feelings by not giving her an invitation. Frank felt it was easier for him and Grant to just suck it up and invite her, even though having her in attendance would feel painful and wrong to both of them. Frank was never good at telling his parents no, however, and this decision was in line with many acquiescences of the past.

How do we clearly communicate boundaries and needs to our significant others, the people closest to us, and ourselves? And why is it so important that we learn how to do so effectively? The reality is that the majority of us who enter into romantic and intimate relationships live in fear. We live in fear that we will be hurt by those we love, that we will come up against something we won't be able to handle, or that we will be taken advantage of by the most significant people in our lives. Add a new and unfamiliar experience like nonmonogamy, or a first-time queer relationship, and you introduce a whole other set of variables and unknowns that generate fear as well.

So what do we do? Our movies and fairy tales tell us that the solution to this is to find the perfect partner: the person who intuitively knows exactly what we are thinking, feeling, and wanting at all times. Some of us try to save ourselves from the pain of the unknown by putting up unyielding barriers around the relationship, or our partners, or ourselves. We give our partners ultimatums and tell them we'll leave if they cross this line or behave in a way we don't like. Conversely, some of us decide we don't want to rock the boat with those to whom we are closest and choose to avoid being too vocal about our wants and needs. We figure our partners (or bosses, family, or friends) will like us more if we just let the little things slide, even if those things secretly make our blood boil. Finally, all that internal strife causes resentment and ultimately a huge blow up. Does any of this sound familiar?

Episode 178, "The Basics of Boundaries" is one of our most downloaded episodes of all time. Why? We believe it's because the vast majority of people have heard of boundaries but are confused as to what they actually are. They are desperate to find better ways to assert themselves and make their values known but haven't found a way that doesn't feel manipulative or controlling. In a landscape full of differing opinions, definitions, and applications for personal boundaries, we wanted to create a clear way to determine what a boundary is, how to utilize and uphold it with others, and how to establish definitions on how boundaries differ from rules or agreements.

What is a boundary?

The concept of personal boundaries started getting hot in therapeutic circles and the self-help world during the 1980s, and it just keeps getting hotter. Multiple books, articles, and blog posts have been published on setting boundaries in relationships, at work, around time, regarding one's body and sexuality, and more. Self-help books and counseling circles love promoting boundaries as the key to success. Setting boundaries is a skill that has entered popular consciousness, and that alone is reason to celebrate!

However, the pop-psych ubiquity of boundaries has resulted in a strange double bind. From the many different sources opining about boundaries, we learn that:

1. Boundaries need to be honored and respected.

Yet, the problem is that:

2. There is no singular, global definition of what boundaries are, what their purpose is, and how they are best utilized in the real world.

This produces a generally agreed-upon sense that "boundaries = good," but understanding the how and why of boundaries is fuzzy. In this context, the word *boundary* gets overused, misconstrued, and made to be a stand-in for other concepts, such as rules, needs, preferences, ultimatums, demands, agreements, expectations, standards, or punishments. Because of this, we see confusing examples of people using the word *boundary* in unclear and ineffective ways, often undermining the very qualities that make boundaries good in the first place:

"My boundary is that you need to be home by ten o'clock tonight."

"I told her I have a boundary about her leaving socks on the floor."

"He broke my boundary when he chose to have unprotected sex with his other partner."

Without a clear sense of what a boundary actually is or how it functions, phrases like these may feel reasonable to some but baffling to others. Even worse, this often encourages people to take something disagreeable or borderline toxic, such as a harsh ultimatum, a demand for control, or a desire to punish the other person, and make it socially acceptable by simply slapping on the "boundary" label. We've seen it happen many times, and it's not cool, kids.

So before we go any further, here is the *Multiamory* definition of a boundary:

A boundary is a guideline, limit, or standard established by you, applied to you, and enforced by you, in order to protect you and preserve your personal values.

That's it! Simple, right? It's different from other definitions floating around out there, so let's take a deeper dive into what this means and why these distinctions are important.

You, you, you, you, you!

You may have noticed that "you" and "your" showed up five times in that short definition. This is because boundaries are all about *you*. This may be the most important aspect of effective boundaries, and we hope that internalizing this truth will help to cut through the fuzziness and confusion around this topic.

You are the one to establish the boundary. You apply it to your own behavior. You enforce it when it's needed to keep you safe and help maintain your integrity. The focus is on you, because the only thing that you can control at the end of the day is *you*. That may be a hard pill to swallow, or it may sound trite because most of us have already heard some version of the serenity prayer:

God grant me the serenity to accept the things I cannot change, courage to change the things I can, and the wisdom to know the difference.

We're not here to tell you that because you're the only thing you can control, that means that other people's behavior and actions shouldn't have any impact. Other people *do* have impact, which is why taking control of your own boundaries is so important. When we construct our boundaries around other people and what we would like them to do, they have a funny habit of transforming into something other than a boundary. Let's look at our previous examples:

> *"My boundary is that you need to be home by ten o'clock tonight."*

This is a request or possibly a rule masquerading as a boundary.

> *"I told her I have a boundary about her leaving socks on the floor."*

This is a preference (potentially a strong preference) masquerading as a boundary.

> *"He broke my boundary when he chose to have unprotected sex with his other partner."*

This is an unmet expectation masquerading as a boundary violation. This could also be a disregarded agreement masquerading as a boundary violation.

Let's make it clear that in your relationships it is not unhealthy to make requests, set up agreements, establish ground rules, or express your preferences and needs. In fact, that's highly encouraged! What's important to remember is that the other person, being an autonomous human being with their own wants, needs, preferences, and behaviors, may bump up against yours by disagreeing, refusing, rejecting, negotiating, or making mistakes. That's where boundaries come in: to make sure that you are able to advocate for *you*.

Rules and Agreements

Before we dive further into boundaries, it's important to briefly define two other words that often get tossed around in relationship communication and especially nonmonogamous education spaces: *rules* and *agreements*. It may feel like we are getting into the nitty-gritty of semantics here, but the intention behind a word is what's most important. We have witnessed the ways in which many people tend to create rules and agreements (sometimes toxic and sometimes not), and those experiences have cemented our ideas on how we describe and educate others on both.

The *Multiamory* stance on rules has generally been: we don't like them. This may seem like a radical approach, because "you have to establish ground rules" is often one of the first pieces of advice that is given whenever two people open up their relationship, decide to embark on an adventurous threesome, or head out to a play party together for the first time. Again, it's easy to think that creating a rule means that you are constructing another protective barrier to make sure you and your partner don't get hurt in the process of a potentially volatile new experience. The problem we've witnessed, however, is that many of the rules that are put in place to save ourselves from pain actually tend to push our partners *away* rather than bring them closer. Besides, what's the overwhelming human reaction when we are told we *can't* do something? It tends to make us want to do the thing that much more.

So what is our definition of a rule?

A rule is a guideline or limit that restricts one person or multiple people's behavior. If the rule is broken, consequences ensue.

That doesn't sound very fun or exciting. And, unlike our definition of a boundary, a rule is something that is done *to* someone else rather than being enacted by yourself and for yourself. Rules not only have potential consequences for the couple or person that is choosing to impose them, but also for many other people in the social or romantic sphere. For example, say a couple opens up their relationship and establishes a rule that they have to be together in the evening for bedtime, every single night, and are not allowed to be over at another partner's house past 11 p.m. This rule not only affects the two people in the initial relationship, but also any other partners they may have. Say a secondary partner gets extremely ill, or has an emergency with an ailing parent, or has to take their dog to the vet at three in the morning. The rule states that you aren't allowed to help or be with that partner past a certain time, and if you do, there's going to be hell to pay. Not only that, but the person who created the rule now has to figure out what the penalty is for breaking it. As we can see, this is a setup for a negative, adversarial dynamic.

We agree with what our friend Cooper S. Beckett, cocreator of the *Life on the Swingset* podcast, says about rules. "Many couples, especially just starting out, will feel that they've lost a sense of 'control' in their relationship. That control, of course, is an illusion, but as they worry they've lost it, they attempt to regain it by building arbitrary rules in. 'No kissing. No sex in our bed. Call before you have sex' et cetera. While I'll admit that for some these serve healthy purposes, for many they're just attempts to retain control at best. At worst, they're argument excuses. I can't state enough, though, that boundaries are perfectly valid, so long as all involved agree without extra pressure." Although Beckett and our earlier example highlight people in multipartner relationships, the same sort of misuse of rules could apply in monogamous, family, or friend situations as well.

An alternative to rules that we find turns partners *toward* each other in collaboration is to create an agreement together. Our definition:

An agreement is a mutual decision between partners that establishes particular behaviors to facilitate trust, accommodate each other's preferences, and provide some predictability as to what they can each expect.

The rule from the earlier example can be easily morphed into an agreement. Maybe one partner has the courage to communicate that they are scared that their partner will leave them if they fall in love with someone else. Maybe what they are really looking for is some real quality time with their partner to remind them how special and important they are to one another. Instead of establishing the rule that they have to be together every night by 11 p.m., they establish an agreement that they will have two date nights a week where they spend meaningful, quality time together.

It might be tempting to simply call a rule an agreement by saying, "We have an *agreement* that we'll always be home by 11 p.m. and never have sleepovers." However, the ideal use of an agreement is to change the focus to positive action rather than limitation. In this example, the agreement creates more connection between the couple by emphasizing what they *can* do to help each other feel good and providing an understanding of what each person wants. Ideally, an agreement allows each partner to feel heard and understood, while also helping to alleviate fear and insecurity that might be causing an issue in the relationship. Again, while the examples above were created through the lens of nonmonogamy, rules and agreements are certainly utilized in monogamous relationships as well.

Rules, agreements, and boundaries are all just different ways we can protect each other and ourselves against what we don't want in our relationships. If we choose to use these tools, the goal is to create them with an understanding of our personal preferences, wants, and needs, and ultimately utilize them in ways that are healthy and kind to our intimate partners. To reiterate, what makes boundaries distinct from agreements and rules is that a boundary serves as a type of *self*-protection rather than relying on another person to do something for you.

Protection Over Punishment

We've talked a lot about boundaries serving as a form of self-protection. But what are we protecting against? Some definitions of boundaries claim that their purpose is to ward off a myriad of things: violation, discomfort, distress, compromise, harm, and so on. We don't like to paint a picture of boundaries being your only weapon against a world that is out to get you. Rather, boundaries can work more like an emergency exit, an ejector seat, or a last line of defense. Understanding and clarifying our boundaries creates a sense of security, and ideally, they will lead us to have relationships and interactions where we rarely have to enforce them. Your preferences, values, and agreements help guide you toward what you *do* want. Your boundaries protect you from what you *don't* want.

"What you don't want" can look many different ways. It could be as simple as wanting to avoid an unnecessarily long phone conversation just as you're getting ready to head out to work. It could be as serious as protecting yourself from physical harm or abuse. It could be private, like choosing to preserve your mental health by abstaining from checking your ex's social media. It could be public, like letting your friends know that you plan on staying away from places that serve alcohol while you're in recovery. Alicia Bunyan Sampson, author and creator of Polyamorous Black Girl, describes how she believes boundaries can be used to protect oneself: "Recognize that boundaries are not at all about our partners but about ourselves and the power that we have over our own decisions. We protect ourselves by examining what we want in relationships, making clear what our limits are, and committing to stepping away whenever our relationships are no longer aligned with what we have chosen for ourselves."

In romantic and other intimate relationships, it can be easy to get spooked by "what you don't want," to the extent that a boundary turns into a punishment for someone else rather than a protection for you. This is when the evil siblings of boundaries rear their ugly heads in the form of demands, ultimatums, and punitive consequences. For example:

"If someone doesn't respond to my text within twenty-four hours, I am going to ignore that person for at least two days the next time they reach out."

"I have told you multiple times that I will break up with you unless you start going to therapy, so you better get on it."

"If we don't take this weekend trip together, I'm not letting you see your other partner until you and I have had sufficient quality time together."

This sort of logic around boundaries is frighteningly common. This doesn't mean that all boundary enforcement is going to be pretty. It is realistic to expect that when you uphold a boundary, especially if you haven't been consistent in doing so before, the other person may experience some bad feelings. The real trouble occurs when the purpose of the boundary becomes about trying to intentionally *cause* those bad feelings as a consequence. While these examples might seem like something only a manipulative person would do, in our experience they rarely happen intentionally. Boundary pitfalls often result from a genuine desire to protect oneself or to make a relationship feel good again. Ebony Hagans, creator of the nonmonogamy advice page Marjani Lane, gives a good reminder: "The reaction to a broken boundary is not more boundaries, rules, and abuse—it is removing yourself from that experience or relationship. That is not a punishment; it's simply you protecting yourself."

While reading the above examples, you may have realized you have a tendency to think about and create boundaries that result in punishing the other person if they are not upheld. If you find that this is the case as we begin to discuss how to create boundaries, try to get curious about your needs and preferences and begin reworking your boundary into something that doesn't require any specific behavioral or emotional change from your partner. At the end of the day, we can't change our partners, no matter what kinds of interventions or ultimatums we throw at them. If you truly believe that something your partner is doing is harmful to you, consider couples counseling, creating an agreement, or take a look at our section "It's Okay to Break Up" in the Extra Tools section.

YourSELF: An exercise for discovering boundaries

Now it's time to discover what your boundaries are. Even after absorbing the information from the first part of this chapter, creating and enforcing your boundaries might seem like a daunting task. At this point, you may not have any clearly established boundaries to use as reference points. As a guidepost, we've created the following exercise to examine your past experiences, use those experiences to begin creating and shaping your personal boundaries, and, finally, prepare to enforce them effectively in your life. To make things simpler, we have created—you guessed it—a handy, dandy acronym to help you remember the steps of this exercise. At the end of the chapter, you'll find a journal prompt to solidify these ideas even further.

When creating your boundaries, all you have to do is remember—it's all about your **SELF**:

Search
Empower
Live it
Follow up

S IS FOR SEARCH

To start, search your memories for past experiences such as arguments, old relationships, or your upbringing, and identify a particular event that conflicts with your values (for more on values, see the Extra Tools section). Look for patterns of upsetting or painful situations that you have found yourself in repeatedly. In these situations, what behaviors from others clash with your own standards of behavior? What about behaviors from yourself? What other aspects from those experiences still cause you pain or hurt? To get some ideas flowing, here are three examples:

- You remember that while you were growing up, your father would constantly interrupt you during discussions. As an adult, you find that when others interrupt you, you often lose your temper and end up lashing out at the offender. Interrupting is something that is incompatible with how you want to treat others and have them treat you, which is why it upsets you so much. Additionally, the habit of losing your temper is something that ends up damaging your relationships and makes discussions more likely to turn into fights.

- You realize you keep ending up overcommitted at work because coworkers ask you to cover for them or help them with tasks more than they offer to help you in return. Initially it may feel like saying yes to these requests fits with your values of being helpful and kind. However, in recognizing this pattern, you realize that saying yes puts you in situations where you are overworked and anxious, causing you to underperform in other areas of your life and ultimately negatively affecting your health and stress levels.

- You notice that when you have conflict with your partner, she resorts to name-calling or bringing up intentionally hurtful things in order to cut you down and deflect attention away from herself. You often attack back or fall apart when those wounds are prodded. In this case, having a partner who says vicious things is in opposition with how you wish to be treated, and your counterattacks are not helpful to either of you.

While brainstorming, it's possible that a list of specific frustrations will immediately come to mind that you want to fix. If this is the case, it's important to keep searching to find underlying patterns that you want to change across the board, rather than focusing on super-specific interactions with a certain person. These acute examples are helpful when getting started, but you will have more success with a boundary that can be applied consistently with multiple people as opposed to just one person. Sometimes a specific boundary may be needed to protect yourself in a particular relationship, but you may find when you dig deeper that there are larger underlying behaviors that stretch into other scenarios.

E IS FOR EMPOWER

Once you have identified a particular recurring pattern and pinpointed how it negatively affects you or your relationships, it's time to take back your power! Start brainstorming what an empowering boundary might look like. Think about what you needed or wanted during these past experiences. What could you have done that might have helped you feel safe, protected, or stable? Remember that your boundary must rely on your own actions and be entirely enforceable by yourself. That's why this is called the "empower" step. Our hope is that after working through this step, you will feel empowered to stop negative patterns in their tracks and use this tool to safeguard against existing vulnerabilities. We will evaluate the effectiveness of your boundary shortly, but for now, focus on thinking of a variety of different ways you could employ a boundary. Come up with multiple options so that you can assess which will work best.

Now, look at the boundary ideas you came up with and evaluate how well they would work in everyday life. How would you use your boundary to protect yourself and your well-being in situations similar to those that caused you to want to create this boundary in the first place? In the case of our previous interrupting example, here are a few different ideas for enforceable boundaries:

- If I notice someone interrupting me, I will stop the conversation and walk away.

- I will no longer have important conversations with people who have a habit of interrupting me.

- If someone interrupts me, I will quickly point it out the first time and let them know I find this unacceptable. If it happens again, I will exit the conversation.

For the example of taking on coworkers' responsibilities, let's look at some more ideas:

- If someone asks me to take on one of their tasks, I will say no.

- I won't answer right away when people ask me to do tasks, so I can check my workload to make sure I have the time to get it done.

- I will help the first person who asks, but I won't take on any more tasks until that one (and my own) are completed.

For the example of name-calling and attacking in arguments, here are a few possibilities:

- If my partner (or anyone) calls me names or directly attacks me, I will stop the argument and leave the room.

- I will not stay in a relationship with someone who resorts to attacking me as a person.

- If my partner calls me names or says something hurtful, I will point it out the first time and tell them how it made me feel. The second time I will exit the conversation.

Before you take your boundary out into the world and move on to the next step, there are three main questions to ask yourself to evaluate how empowering your boundary may be:

1. Is it realistically possible to enforce a boundary in the way I envisioned?
For example, would walking out of the room work in every situation, or would there be moments where it might be difficult or impossible to do that? What happens if someone keeps trying to engage with me after I tell them no?

2. Would I actually do it?
In practice, you may have a hard time enforcing the boundary you have created. The boundary may require you to be in a calm emotional state, but when a challenging situation arises, you're upset and frustrated. You may find adjusting the boundary to happen earlier, before you get emotionally activated, will yield the result you wanted. In other scenarios, you might ask yourself, "Are the consequences of this boundary too big for me to enforce? Would I stop a conversation or leave a relationship if it came to it?"

Which leads us to the final question:

3. Can I enforce this boundary consistently across all situations? Remember, a boundary is most effective when it is nonnegotiable for yourself. For example, you might take a break from

an argument with your partner if they raise their voice, but when your boss does it, you stay in the room. In that case, you might need to adjust the boundary to be more specific, or you may just need to work up the courage to actually enforce the boundary with your boss. Ultimately, you are the one making the boundaries, and you are the person who will enforce them. For best results, evaluate your situation and make choices that are extensions of you and your values.

L IS FOR LIVE IT

Now is the time to put your boundary into practice and live it in your daily life. In some cases, this may also be the time to tell a partner or a friend about a particular boundary and let them know how you will enforce it in the future if the time comes. You might tell a partner, "Just a heads-up, I really don't respond well when someone raises their voice, so if either of us starts yelling while we are arguing, I am going to leave the room and stop the conversation until we both can calm down. I will wait to restart our discussion until we can come back together with less emotional intensity."

When you let those closest to you know about a boundary, it increases the chances they'll be more understanding once it gets utilized. They may still be resistant or defensive in the moment, but by reducing the element of surprise, you may set yourself up for more productive conversations later. This can also be an effective way to "recruit" loved ones as backup in moments where you need to enforce your boundary with someone else. Recruiting the support of friends can go a long way when trying to enforce a difficult boundary.

Alternately, since your boundary is personal to you and only enforceable by you, it may not always be necessary to make a big announcement. Posting a notice in the break room that you will automatically refuse all requests to cover someone else's shift could backfire. As long as you feel firm and clear with yourself about your boundary and how to operationalize it, you don't necessarily need to stress about issuing a boundary press release to everyone in your life. However you approach it, the most important part of this step is to enforce the boundary to the best of your ability, see how it feels, and assess how it affects your relationships. You might even try keeping a boundary journal to track how well your boundaries are working (or not working).

F IS FOR FOLLOW UP

Once you have lived with your boundary for a little while, it is time to follow up with yourself and see if it's time to adjust and tweak. This is where a boundary journal can come in handy! You may realize you can better uphold your boundary if you make a tiny adjustment, or you may need to go back to the drawing board and change it entirely. Here are some follow-up questions to try on:

- What happened the last time I enforced this boundary? Did anything surprising happen?

- What feelings came up for me when I had to enforce this boundary?

- What reactions did I get from the other person? Were they shocked? Understanding? Frustrated?

- Have I been able to enforce this boundary across multiple situations and relationships?

- Is this boundary too restrictive, too general, too rigid, or too porous?

- Does this boundary rely on a behavior change from someone else or some other external change out of my control?

- Is this boundary even necessary anymore?

- What actionable steps am I going to take moving forward to make this boundary more effective?

Revisit the follow-up step periodically, especially if it is a boundary that comes up often. You may require numerous reworkings of your boundary over a period of time or the course of your entire life! Think of this as entering the "longitudinal study" phase of understanding which boundaries work best for you. Each time a new person comes into your life, your life circumstances change, you stumble on the need for a new boundary, or you uncover fresh insight about yourself and your relationships, use it as an opportunity to follow up on your boundaries once again.

Boundaries in Real Life

Hopefully by now, you are pumped about boundaries, and you're ready to create and try them out! The truth is the real-life application of boundaries can look many, many different ways. It would be easier if we had a social script that made it acceptable to simply say, "This is my boundary, and this is how I will enforce it if necessary." But because it is rarely that simple or straightforward, we've listed a few real-world examples to showcase the many different shapes that boundaries can take.

THE INTERNAL BOUNDARY

You are feeling some deep NRE (new relationship energy) for a new partner. You sent a text to them what feels like hours ago, and they still haven't responded. (It was actually only eight minutes ago.) You can't keep still, and you stop what you're doing every few minutes to check for a read receipt (still no). As thrilling as the new connection is, getting their response isn't urgent, and you're finding yourself frustrated by being unable to focus while trying to spend some quality time with your family. You value being focused and present for quality time with them, and this frantic phone checking is getting in the way of that. You decide that you're going to protect yourself from the distraction by stashing your phone in your car's glove box for the rest of the evening.

THE MENTAL NOTE

You have found yourself in a conversation about workplace politics with a friend at a party. Even though you agree with most of what they're saying, you were looking forward to being able to disconnect from work and catch up with your friend. However, they are speaking about something they are passionate about, and you don't want to be dismissive. You muster up all your friend powers in order to continue offering a listening ear for now, but you do make a mental note: when the two of you meet up later this week for lunch, you'll take action to steer the conversation away from work, and you'll speak up if your friend keeps on insisting on taking it there.

THE NO THANKS

After date number three, a new partner started unloading on you about their ex. Or, at least, you're pretty sure it's an ex. This person was open about the fact that they still occasionally hook up with their ex, even though they called it quits months ago. There seems to still be a lot of unfinished business, and you are hearing all about the continuing drama. In fact, you're starting to feel like this person is turning you into a therapist for unpacking their relationship issues. You are not a fan, especially since you've already been burned by having a partner's outside relationship troubles spill onto you. You know that this is going to be a huge drain on your energy and emotions, so you finally decide to enforce a boundary: "I'm going to take a step back from developing our relationship so that you can have some time and space to figure things out with your ex. We can still stay in touch, but I won't participate in conversations that are only about your relationship problems."

As an aside, when embarking on new relationships, having early boundary discussions can prove to be a hugely beneficial practice. "It's so important to have some baseline boundaries when meeting new potential partners," says Erin Tillman, sex educator and dating empowerment coach. "While it's up to each individual to decide the importance of specific kinds of boundaries, it could be extremely helpful to have a general idea about the things you consider to be nonnegotiable or deal breakers. These early make-or-break nonnegotiable boundaries could include differing relationship styles, mismatched communication style or frequency of communication, quality time requirements or limitations, or even political leanings. Having a general idea of what specific things could be a conflict for you and someone else could save you both time, energy, and potential heartache."

EMILY SAYS

At one point in my late twenties, I was working no fewer than three different restaurant jobs, doing personal assistant work, and auditioning for voice and acting gigs in Los Angeles. All this work was happening in addition to creating and producing the *Multiamory* podcast every week with Jase and Dedeker! Was I so strapped for cash that I needed to have so many jobs? Negative. I just didn't want to say no to the people who asked me to work for them.

It didn't take long for my relationship and my quality of life to suffer because I was working so much. While my partner had a normal nine-to-five, I sometimes wouldn't be home until 11 p.m. Our schedules almost never overlapped, so my day off never seemed to coincide with my partner's. The grueling hours and stress were cause for a lot of unhappiness and exhaustion during this time.

Then one day a coworker noticed me finishing up side work at one of the restaurants during the end of my shift. I was tired and irritable at the prospect of having to work the morning shift at a different restaurant the next day. The coworker knew about all the things I was trying to pack into my life. They looked at me appraisingly and asked me a simple question: "Emily, what are you trying to prove?"

It was like a bolt of lightning hit me. What the hell was I trying to prove? I'm a hard worker, people seem to like me, and they would probably understand if I needed to change my day-to-day life in order to do what was best for me (and if they didn't, fuck 'em). So the next day, I put in my two weeks' notice at one of the restaurants. Six months later, I did the same at another. I significantly cut my hours at my personal assistant job and changed my schedule so I only worked during the day and had at least one day off every weekend to spend with my partner. In order to save myself from myself, I put a boundary in place to limit the amount of time I spent engaging with jobs I didn't need or enjoy. It made a tremendous difference in my quality of life.

THE RESTATEMENT

You're excited to be moving into a new apartment, and your dad has come over to help with the move. At one point, he looks around the place and turns to you. "This looks like a pretty nice place. How much did you have to put down for your deposit?" You immediately stiffen. There is a long history of uncomfortable money conversations with your dad, often filled with judgment and unsolicited advice. It finally reached a breaking point a few months ago, when you got up the courage to establish a boundary with him: "I will only discuss my personal finances with my partner, with whom I share a bank account." Him asking this question suggests that either he's forgotten your boundary or he doesn't take it seriously. You feel hesitant, but you take a breath and say, "I'm going to remind you that I'm choosing to discuss money stuff only with my partner." You see his jaw tense a little bit in annoyance, but to your surprise he says, "All right, fair enough," and gets back to unpacking boxes.

THE EJECTOR SEAT

For this example, here's Dedeker's real-life story:

DEDEKER SAYS

I had been dating Sam for about a year when he dropped a bomb: he wanted to get back together with his ex-girlfriend, who was not a fan of nonmonogamy and certainly not a fan of me. Sam still wanted to be in a relationship with both of us and was struggling to figure out how to rectify the situation. He finally came to me one day with a proposal.

"I talked it over with her, and she told me that she's okay with you being in the picture as long as you and I aren't having sex. So, we can still be together and be affectionate, we just won't have sex."

You can imagine how well that went over with me. It was less about the sex itself and more about the feeling of betrayal that a decision like this had been made without my input or buy-in whatsoever. For a long time, I had highly valued practicing nonhierarchical and noncoercive polyamory, which to me meant respecting the autonomy of myself and others by not allowing one person or one relationship to make unilateral decisions about another person or relationship. I wanted to be in a relationship with Sam, but this new situation directly clashed with my values.

I wish I could say that I immediately asserted my boundaries and everything ended up happily ever after, but it was a bit messier than that. My first move was to put up a "boundary" of asking for two weeks without contact in order to have some time and space to process this. This was only a half-baked boundary. On the one hand, it did protect my emotional bandwidth by buying some time, but to be honest, I was also using it as a punishment. There was a part of me deep down that was hoping that because I put up this punishing boundary, Sam would feel enough regret and hurt that he would realize the error of his ways.

After two weeks' time, Sam's position didn't budge, and neither had mine. It was then I realized that it was time for an actual boundary on my part. I knew I couldn't be in a relationship under these terms, and so I told him that. Then I had to make the difficult effort to enforce that by taking myself out of the relationship. No "breaks," no revisiting, no plans to reconnect or try again later down the road.

It fucking sucked.

After all was said and done, I was overwhelmed by how bittersweet it felt to enforce my own boundaries in such a big way. I had to deal with the grief that comes with the loss of a relationship, but that pain was mixed with a strange sense of victory. It could have been easy to compromise too much, begrudgingly agreeing to terms that didn't support my values just for the sake of keeping this person in my life. But my boundary had saved me from that heartache. I put up a boundary. I dealt with the pain and upset, and I survived. That experience alone has supercharged the confidence I have in my own boundaries.

Troubleshooting: Obstacles to Effective Boundaries

Boundaries are a deep, complex, far-reaching topic. It's difficult to troubleshoot boundary issues, since it so often depends on context, individual history, and personality. However, there are some common themes. Many problems related to boundaries are the result of the many obstacles that can get in the way of us effectively setting or enforcing our own boundaries. Here are just a few:

- Being afraid of pushing people away

- The risk that someone may dislike or react strongly to your boundary

- Fear of missing out on an experience or opportunity, even if it will come at a great cost to your well-being

- Being raised in a family that discouraged boundary setting

- Living in a culture that discourages boundary setting

- Not wanting to feel exposed and vulnerable

- Having a past experience of being punished, gaslit, hurt, or abused for trying to enforce a boundary

- Having a past experience of someone else's boundaries being weaponized against you

- Having a past experience of your boundaries being ignored or steamrolled

- Being unsure what your personal boundaries are, how to express them, or how to enforce them

- Fear of being seen as stubborn, mean, selfish, boring, a bad partner, a bad employee, a bad friend, a bad child/parent/family member, or a bad person

- Fear of rejection

It can feel like the deck is stacked against you. Boundaries are important, but that doesn't mean they are always easy to maintain. The culture you grew up in or the identities that you hold can make this even more difficult. "We all have a formula for what we're willing to put up with when it comes to living the life we want to live," shares Kevin Patterson, author of *Love's Not Color Blind*. "Sometimes that means brushing off a microaggression that would normally upset you in order to engage in an activity you're excited about. Sometimes that means divorcing yourself from a group altogether and/or starting your own. It's a constant struggle to protect our sanity, to maintain our personal respect, and to live our best, most fulfilling lives. It's a concern that dominant groups and identities don't have and are largely oblivious to."

A TWO-WAY STREET

Many boundary problems can be related to the countless obstacles that can get in the way of us effectively understanding and acknowledging *other people's* boundaries. The way we juggle our own boundaries along with the boundaries of others can offer some interesting clues. If you're finding it difficult to understand or honor other people's boundaries, it is likely you may have similar struggles with your own boundaries.

These are just some of the obstacles that can make it difficult to respect other people's boundaries:

- Thinking that you know better about what the other person wants

- Disagreeing with the stated or perceived reason behind the boundary

- Feeling rejected or embarrassed

- Failing to ask about the other person's boundaries or failing to get enough information to fully understand their boundaries

- Having past experience of someone else's boundaries being weaponized against you

- Not even realizing that the person has a boundary

- Projecting your own boundaries (or lack thereof) onto the other person

- Taking the boundary enforcement personally, or making someone else's boundary mean something negative about yourself

- A history of interacting with someone who has not expressed or enforced any boundaries until now

- Fear of missing out on an experience or opportunity, even if it will come at a great cost to the other person's well-being

- Being raised in a family that discourages honoring the boundaries of others

- Being raised in a culture that discourages honoring the boundaries of others

It is easy to think that anyone who violates or pushes against a boundary is a bad, villainous person. The sad reality is that all of us are guilty of this behavior in big and small ways. Dedeker got a wake-up call about this even in a fairly benign situation:

DEDEKER SAYS

I was at a workshop a few years ago where we were exploring giving and receiving pleasurable touch. Because everyone was paired up with strangers, it was only nonsexual touch, with a heavy emphasis on consent. For one exercise, I was paired up with a woman that I didn't know. I asked if I could give her a foot massage. She hesitated before saying, "Um, no, it's just that I'm wearing a pair of shoes that make my feet really sweaty and smelly . . ."

Before she could say anything else, I rushed in—"Oh, that's okay! I don't mind"—and I proceeded to settle on the floor, ready to dive into the massage. She looked at me and said a little more firmly, "I'd rather not get a foot massage, thank you."

It was at that moment I realized that I had tried to steamroll this woman's boundary without even thinking! As I thought about it afterward, I was amazed by just how slippery these scenarios can be. In an attempt at being nice and caring and accommodating, I was being anything but, by failing to actually listen to what she said. And this was a pretty low-stakes scenario with a stranger; there have probably been hundreds of times that I have done something similar with people that I care about.

The story above illustrates how boundaries can be accidentally violated even when we are trying to be kind, caring, or understanding of others. It's an important lesson to remember and a reminder to give yourself and your partner some grace when first learning about and implementing boundaries into your relationships.

TURN A POROUS BOUNDARY INTO SOMETHING CONCRETE

Our opening story with Frank and Grant showed a porous, unclear definition of a personal boundary, coupled with a need to please generous family members. Porous boundaries are often associated with those of us who tend to fawn as a response to trauma (for more on fawning and trauma responses, see the Extra Tools section). These boundaries may happen as a result of having difficulty saying no, fear of rejection, or an overwhelming desire to please others, among many other factors.

Frank didn't want to put himself or the man he loves in an uncomfortable position at their wedding, yet the pull to please his parents was overriding the wishy-washy boundary he had put in place. Even though he knew it was important to him that he and Grant felt happy and secure at their wedding, he didn't have any actionable recourse to follow through with those sentiments. Similarly, you may have discovered when you were doing the SELF exercise that you tend to create porous and difficult-to-execute boundaries. If this is the case, it's important to work through the underlying reasons why you struggle with upholding your boundaries. Consult with a friend or therapist, break out your journal, or do some self-analysis. You may find it helpful to create a few modest boundaries with less dire ramifications and practice getting better at enforcing those before you move on to bigger, more consequential boundaries.

Once Frank had spent some time practicing implementing less significant boundaries in his life, he was ready to tackle this important situation again. He decided that being firm in his enforcement of this boundary was a necessary solution. Instead of allowing his parents to dictate the course of his wedding day, which might leave both him and Grant vulnerable to microaggressions and insults from his aunt, he needed to be ultra-clear on how he would enforce this boundary. Communicating your boundary to another person can sound a variety of different ways. In this instance, *internally* establishing what would happen if Frank's parents chose to disregard the boundary and invite his aunt to the wedding, and then *externally* communicating this as nonnegotiable to his parents, was essential. After listening to *Multiamory* Episode 178, The Basics of Boundaries, and getting support from Grant, Frank was finally able to uphold his boundary and have a straightforward discussion with his parents:

> *"I am not going to allow homophobic people to attend the most important day of my life. I am choosing to keep myself and my partner safe by not inviting my aunt to the wedding. You may not approve, but this is nonnegotiable for me. If you choose to disregard this, I will have to call my aunt and uninvite her to the wedding."*

With this statement, Frank was clear in his communication, established his expectations, and let his parents know that he would take action to ensure that he and his partner remain safe. Again, this is a personal boundary to protect himself, not a chance to punish his parents! He clearly communicated the action that will be taken if the boundary is crossed, in order to protect himself and his partner. The wedding went off without a hitch!

Homework: SELF

To bring it all home, use the SELF exercise to create your own boundaries.

1. Search: Write down at least three meaningful past experiences such as volatile arguments, challenging old relationships, or your upbringing and family of origin, and then identify particular moments that felt contrary to your standards of behavior or how you want to be treated by another person. In these situations, what behaviors from others clash with your own standards of behavior? What about behaviors from yourself? What other aspects from those experiences still cause you pain or hurt? Try to identify and write down recurring patterns of behavior from these meaningful experiences and how they might be affecting your relationships.

2. Empower: Begin brainstorming what a boundary might look like. Remember that an empowering boundary must be entirely enforceable by you. Write down one to three enforceable boundaries for each of the scenarios you uncovered in the search step. Then, evaluate those boundaries and write down your responses to the following in your journal:

1. Is it realistically possible to enforce this boundary in the way I've envisioned?

2. Would I actually do it?

3. Can I enforce this consistently across situations?

3. Live It: Go apply your boundary in real life. Figure out if you need to inform people about your new boundary, but remember that in some situations, it may be all right to just keep it to yourself. Keep a journal of your experiences.

4. Follow Up: After trying it out for some time, take stock of your experience and see if the boundary needs some tweaking or adjusting. You may realize right away that you need to make changes for yourself, or you may need to gather more data and continue to practice your boundary. Run through these follow-up questions:

- What happened the last time I enforced this boundary? Did anything surprising happen?

- What feelings came up for me when I had to enforce this boundary?

- What reactions did I get from the other person? Were they shocked? Understanding? Frustrated?

- Have I been able to enforce this boundary across multiple situations and relationships?

- Is this boundary too restrictive, too general, too rigid, or too porous?

- Does this boundary rely on a behavior change from someone else or some other external change out of my control?

- Is this boundary even necessary anymore?

- What actionable steps am I going to take moving forward to make this boundary more effective?

Remember to revisit the follow-up step and the SELF exercise again and again as your life circumstances change and as new relationships develop.

Takeaways

- A boundary is a guideline, limit, or standard established by you, applied to you, and enforced by you, in order to protect you and preserve your personal values.

- A rule is a guideline or limit that restricts one or multiple people's behavior. If the rule is broken, consequences ensue.

- An agreement is a mutual decision between partners that establishes particular behaviors to facilitate trust, accommodate each other's preferences, and provide some predictability as to what they can each expect.

- Your boundaries protect you from what you *don't* want. Your preferences, values, and agreements help guide you toward what you *do* want.

- The goal is that you will develop relationships where you rarely need to enforce boundaries, since they are meant to be a last line of defense.

- A boundary is not a punishment for another person, but it is there to act as a way to help you protect yourself.

- When creating your boundaries, all you have to do is remember, it's all about your **SELF**:

> Search
> Empower
> Live it
> Follow up

- Brainstorm the things that are important to you and what has affected your behavior and relationships in the past and create a boundary that will protect you from pain and hurt that you have previously experienced. Use your SELF to aid in this process! Be clear on what the actionable enforcement of your boundary will look like. Use it when necessary. If it doesn't work out, adjust and repeat.

- Communicate with your partner about your boundary and why it is important that you personally enforce it. Or be mindful of situations when it may be best to keep your boundary to yourself.

- Be aware of the boundaries of others, listen well, and ask questions if you are unsure. Give yourself some grace when you inevitably screw up enforcing your boundaries or adhering to the boundaries of others.

For more information, check out *Multiamory* Episode 178, "The Basics of Boundaries" and Episode 227, "Rules vs. Agreements feat. Boundaries."

CHAPTER 6

Repair SHOP:
Mend and
Prevent Conflict

Lyla and Kevin had already been arguing for hours. Lyla had agreed to let Kevin know if she was going to be coming home later than expected from her date with her other partner, Sarah. She did send a text, but it was after she'd already been out two hours later than when she said she'd be home. Kevin had gone through a whole gamut of emotions—restless, nervous, afraid, annoyed, angry—by the time Lyla walked in the door. It was late, but the two proceeded to stay up even later butting heads.

"You said that you would let me know if you were staying out later than planned. I can't believe you would find it so easy to disregard a simple courtesy that we both agreed to. You're so self-centered!" Kevin ranted.

But Lyla went on the defensive. "I did what we agreed to, just not at a time that *you* wanted it to happen. I don't think this is that big of a deal, and you're getting much more worked up about it than you need to," she insisted.

After going in circles numerous times, the pair finally reached a point of physical, mental, and emotional exhaustion.

"I can't talk about this anymore," Lyla sighed as she crawled under the covers.

Kevin stared at her, feeling a new wave of anger and fear. Too drained to keep the dialogue going, Kevin also collapsed into bed, turning his back to his partner.

The next day was tense, as the two largely avoided each other. By that evening, they were each calm enough to exchange some small talk about dinner plans. Lyla initiated a cuddle on the couch, and both of them inwardly felt relieved to be connected again. Kevin still felt like he hadn't been heard, and Lyla still felt hurt by Kevin's criticism, but that relief felt so good that neither of them really wanted to revisit their communication breakdown.

This was the status quo for a couple weeks until Lyla was headed out on a date again. Leading up to Lyla's departure, both were quiet, unable to avoid thinking about the previous blowup.

As she headed out the door, Kevin said stiffly, "Try being a little more considerate of me this time."

Lyla instantly felt pangs of the hurt from before. Instead of sharing, she simply said, "Sure," and swung the door shut with enough force to make a point. Even though they had reconnected and let their previous fight pass, seeds had already been planted for the next cycle of blowups.

When Repair Is Absent

Fights and arguments are inevitable in close relationships, and while they may be cathartic, they are often deeply uncomfortable and sometimes traumatic. When the bridge between yourself and your partner gets broken, even from a small disagreement, it can bring up deep-seated feelings of abandonment, confusion, and disorientation. It is the feeling of separation from our partner that can be the most upsetting, and we desperately want to be close again. Repair is the essential ingredient that catalyzes conflict into understanding, empathy, and action that restores closeness and improves the relationship over time. Our human instincts and desires set us up to *want* to repair and reconnect, but the actual undertaking of repair can be much more difficult. Unfortunately, a lack of repair after one argument can make it even harder to repair in the next one, and a chronic cycle is born.

Here are a few of the problems that can arise from a chronic lack of repair:

PROGRESS AND RESOLUTION COME TO A HALT.

This may be redundant, but when you don't repair, *stuff doesn't get repaired.* You and your partner may leave a fight with more clarity about how the other person feels, but all that can be for naught if there isn't proactive, positive change attached to it. At worst, you may leave a fight with the assumption that your partner understands exactly what to do to make things better next time, only to be disappointed when they don't do it.

RESENTMENT BUILDS UP.

Resentment arises when we feel that we've been mistreated or that someone has been unfair. An unrepaired fight can hit on both fronts: your partner's aggressive behavior or harsh criticism may feel like mistreatment, and your partner leaving the fight without truly listening or understanding your viewpoint can feel extremely unfair. If this is left unaddressed, bitterness creeps in, which can affect not only your mood but also how you see and treat your partner on a day-to-day basis.

NEGATIVITY BECOMES THE DEFAULT.

There can be a curious Jekyll-and-Hyde dynamic that arises in relationships. You and your partner may be warm, kind, and affectionate most of the time, only to turn nasty when conflict arises. The memory of a partner's raised voice, angry look, or mean comment doesn't magically disappear as soon as the waters have calmed again. Those experiences feed into your mental narrative about your partner. If bad behavior during fights has never been acknowledged or mended, that narrative turns negative and stays negative. Soon, you come to *expect* interactions with your partner to be unpleasant, setting the groundwork for conflict avoidance and preemptive defensiveness and hostility.

VULNERABILITY AND AUTHENTICITY DISAPPEAR.

When we are exposed to the constant discomfort and pain of unresolved conflict, it takes a toll. If you don't feel seen, heard, or understood, on top of feeling wounded by your partner's words or actions, it activates our self-protective instincts. It becomes that much more important to conceal your true thoughts and feelings, because showing your tender, fearful side becomes too much of a risk. Vulnerability is the gateway to intimacy, but hurtful arguments left unrepaired act like bricks blocking off the entry.

PRECIOUS TIME IS LOST.

Time spent in a state of disrepair is time wasted. It's important to clarify that the time you and your partner have *intentionally* dedicated to taking a pause and calming down before coming back to a discussion is different. What we're referring to as wasted time is the long, drawn-out holding pattern that occurs when the energy of a fight has petered out but the upset feelings have not, leading one or both of you to sulk, avoid each other, give the cold shoulder, or get sucked back into the same fight over and over again.

What gets in the way of repair

Not everyone avoids repair. Many people do understand the importance of processing a breakdown, both on their own and with a partner. Unfortunately, attempts at repair and processing can often go awry, sometimes escalating into a blowout that is even worse than the original incident. These are some common bad habits that can derail a good attempt at repair:

FIGHTING OVER THE NARRATIVE

"You walked in the door in a huff and immediately stomped off to the bedroom, then—"

"No, I did not! I asked how your day was first."

"No, you didn't. You didn't even look at me! You only asked me about my day after I followed you into the room."

"You have it all wrong!"

And so on and so on.

It is easy to make the mistake of thinking that processing a fight equals coming to an agreed-upon narrative of what happened during the fight or why the fight happened in the first place. While it feels good to get on the same page as your partner, the reality is that this often creates a power struggle. Each of us is cognitively biased to believe that our version of the story is the correct one, and we just need to get our partner to see how they have completely mistaken what happened. The problem is that the other person is usually thinking the same thing!

This is one of the easiest ways to get drawn back into the fight without making any real progress. It immediately becomes necessary to win by dominating with our "correct" version of events. Fighting over the narrative sets us up to be combative rather than collaborative from the very start. Dr. Stan Tatkin, author of *Wired for Love*, calls this "blah-blah-blah" warfare: all words, no substance.

FOCUSING ON UNSOLVABLE PROBLEMS

A 2019 study published in *Family Process* found that happy couples approach arguments in a different way. Not only do happy couples differ in *how* they resolve and process conflict, but also in *what* topics they choose to even discuss in the first place. Researchers found that happy couples more often chose to discuss topics that felt solvable, rather than focusing on topics that were difficult to resolve or completely unsolvable.

Determining the difference between a solvable and unsolvable problem is the real kicker. It's not quite as easy as categorizing certain topics as solvable and others as unsolvable. It may be easier to explain by example:

Solvable problem: Whether to go to your best friend's birthday dinner by yourself or with your partner.

Unsolvable problem: How to get your partner to suddenly become extroverted enough that they'll happily commit to going to dinner, drinks, and the karaoke afterparty as well.

Solvable problem: How to afford a replacement for the refrigerator that just broke down.

Unsolvable problem: Determining who has a better approach to handling money and who got us into this mess in the first place.

Solvable problem: How to arrange childcare so that your partner can go to synagogue once a week.

Unsolvable problem: Convincing your partner that their religious beliefs are garbage and not worth the effort.

Solvable problem: Making decisions about which safer sex practices make sense and feel reasonable for you and your partner.

Unsolvable problem: Making decisions about whose sexual risk tolerance is superior.

You might notice a running theme. The unsolvable problems tend to be associated with differences in personality, identity, beliefs, and core needs. Gottman Institute research indicates that as much as 69 percent of conflict in relationships is related to fundamental differences, which they have labeled as "perpetual problems." A good way to tell if a problem is related to fundamental differences is to ask yourself, "Would this problem go away if my partner just erased this one annoying part of their personality?" If the answer is "Yes, they really need to shape up!" then it's likely you have an unsolvable problem on your hands.

The terminology is pretty doom-and-gloom. Calling a problem "perpetual" and "unsolvable" does not exactly inspire hope. However, it's futile to deny the reality of deal breakers. There may be foundational aspects of your partner that are incompatible with who you are and what you want, to the extent that the relationship may not be a good fit. And that's okay—as always, it's okay to leave a relationship that is not working (more on that in the Extra Tools section).

However, don't subscribe to the myth that it's possible to

find a relationship with zero incompatibilities. Dan Wile, therapist and author of *After the Fight*, says, "When choosing a long-term partner, you will inevitably be choosing a particular set of unsolvable problems that you'll be grappling with for the next ten, twenty, or fifty years."

When you take stock of the differences between yourself and your partner, do they feel like insurmountable obstacles? Or can you both find pathways to compromise while still making each other feel fundamentally accepted and loved?

JUMPING IN TOO QUICKLY

Looking at the scary list of all the bad things that can happen if there's a chronic lack of repair may lead you to think that repair needs to happen as quickly as humanly possible. This is a common tendency among those of us who have a more anxious attachment style or who tend to be the "pursuers" in relationship conflict. The drive to reconnect and feel safe again is strong and can lead to rushing into a repair process before it's the right time (check out the sections in Extra Tools on attachment styles and Demon Dance Battles for more information about pursuit and withdrawal patterns in relationships).

When is the right time? When you and your partner are physiologically calm. The emphasis here is on *physiological* calm—your heart rate, breathing, and muscles are at or close to the state they would be for you on a normal, uneventful day. The key is waiting until you're no longer in survival mode. That jittery, fight-or-flight sensation makes it nearly impossible to listen compassionately or communicate clearly. This does not mean you have to wait until you are no longer angry, sad, anxious, unsettled, or any other emotion. You can have a body and nervous system that is calm or close to calm while still feeling full of emotions. It can be helpful to recognize what your survival response tends to look like, and you can find more about that in the section on fight, flight, freeze, and fawn in the Extra Tools section.

It's difficult to prescribe exactly how much time to let pass between the end of a fight and the beginning of a repair. Many therapists recommend a minimum of twenty minutes to a maximum of twenty-four hours. If you and your partner are able to walk away from a fight and still be civil and kind to each other, you may be able to wait even longer before processing what happened. The fights and arguments section of a RADAR (see Chapter 7) could be a good time for this!

It isn't recommended to put off repairs for too long. However, in Dedeker's work with clients, she has seen people make fantastic repairs even weeks, months, or years after the original incident. At the end of the day, having an ongoing practice of repair is what matters. "We all mess up, even with the people we love the most. What makes a stable, loving relationship is the ability to move compassionately through disharmony, not the ability to avoid it (which is actually impossible)," says Libby Sinback, relationship coach and host of the podcast *Making Polyamory Work*. "That process of getting from disharmony back to harmony is *everything*. Feeling like you can mess up with a partner and not lose the relationship makes the relationship feel strong and the people in it feel secure. And while coming up with solutions to problems can be helpful, the most important part of making up with a partner is that everyone feels seen and heard and held with respect."

At this point, you probably have some questions about what even goes into making an effective repair. You may be wondering:

1. Is it just saying, "I'm sorry"?

2. Does it have to involve makeup sex?

3. Is *Multiamory* about to drop an acronym on me?

Answers: 1) No, 2) Definitely not, and 3) Heck yes.

Repair SHOP: An Introduction

Welcome to the Repair SHOP—a four-step process that you and your partner can go through once you are ready to process a fight or argument. Repair SHOP was inspired by research from the Gottman Institute's Love Lab on repair attempts, the aftermath of a fight, and "regrettable instances" in couples. This process works best once you have both had a chance to cool off and feel physiologically ready to reconnect with your partner. Going through these steps will not only help you both to repair your connection after a specific fight, but it will also give you deeper insights into each other's inner worlds and help you to avoid future conflicts as well.

If the fight you had was new and felt unconnected to other issues, then the SHOP process might be quick and will help to ensure that whatever you were fighting about doesn't become a recurring problem. On the other hand, if this feels like a persistent fight or has connections to other recurring conflicts in your relationship, then this process may take more time in order to allow each of you to feel heard and to facilitate compassion.

One key to a successful relationship Repair SHOP is both parties having an understanding of the framework and of the principles behind it. While some of the tools in this book, like the Triforce of Communication (Chapter 2), can be effective even if the other person has no idea what it is, we have found that this tool in particular works best if both of you approach it with some comprehension of how it works, what you are trying to accomplish, and the importance of the process.

Repair SHOP is not about getting a second chance to prove that you were right in an argument. It won't help you change fundamental aspects of your partner's personality. Nor will you be forcing yourself to give half-hearted apologies in order to keep the peace. The ultimate goal here is to develop a better understanding of one another and to clarify intentions or actions that will help to avoid future bitterness, resentment, and frustration. And yes, because it's *Multiamory*, you get a fun acronym that will guide you through each step.

Here's the road map of what to expect, with in-depth explanations of each step to follow:

SHOP

Stories
History
Ownership
Prevention

While engaging in Repair SHOP, you and your partner will go through each step together and take turns talking and listening. Depending on how each of you is feeling after the argument, this process may be challenging, so be sure you are both showing up with your best communication tools and an underlying desire to connect and care for each other. Ideally, the person who is taking a turn listening should not interrupt their partner and instead should work to understand the experience and the emotions of the other person. Remember, the two of you are together because you love each other and want each other to be happy in the relationship, so taking the time to set aside your ego is key.

S IS FOR STORIES

The first step to repair is to better understand each other's experience of the conflict. The power of this step comes from the realization that each of us has our own unique viewpoint of any event that we are a part of. Even if two people witness the same event, they will each notice slightly different things, and their past experiences, knowledge, and beliefs will influence how they feel about what they are seeing. Generally, when you're in the middle of a fight, you are focused on your own experience and may believe your interpretation of events is universally true for everyone else who was involved. Often this belief creates a majority of the conflict, and you may each try to convince the other person that your perception of reality is the correct one.

For this first Repair SHOP step, in an effort to better understand each other, take turns telling your story of what happened during the fight. Be mindful of focusing on your own experience without trying to dictate to the other person what they were feeling or intending to do during the disagreement. For example, "When you got up and walked out of the room, I felt like you had given up on me, and I was scared of being abandoned" is better than "You gave up on me and abandoned me by walking out of the room right when you knew it would hurt the most." It can take some practice to learn to express your feelings without phrases like, "You made me feel _____," so take your time and be mindful during this specific step. This is a good opportunity to use your best communication skills and employ some techniques like nonviolent communication, clean talk, or I-messages (check out the Extra Tools section for more information on each of these tools). Try to gently help your partner understand your experience of what happened. How did you feel? Were you sad, angry, worried, lonely, ashamed, or defensive?

As the listener, your job is to pay attention and listen without adding any corrections or interjections. Understand that you each experienced a different but equally valid reality during your fight. The purpose of this step isn't to rehash the argument or to clarify who was right or wrong. The only goal in this step is to listen and understand that your partner may have experienced a different truth from your own, with different meanings, perceptions, and emotions.

This can be a challenge! Listening to your partner's version of events may cause you to internally scream, "They're mistaken!! They have it all wrong!!" But once you get the hang of it, it can be a transformative and eye-opening experience. Therapist and author Martha Kauppi shares her take on how easy it can be to get bogged down by our own personal perceptions of what occurred during a disagreement: "When you have a stressful interaction, your brain records a unique and personal perception of what happened, from your own unique perspective, which is informed by the entirety of your own personal history. In other words, perceptions are as unique as fingerprints. Everyone's fingerprint is equally valid. Let go of the desire to square up your perceptions of history, and instead focus on understanding one another's experiences, perceptions, and the meanings each of you made of whatever happened. From there, you will be better able to understand and even empathize with an experience that is very different from your own."

This step on its own can sometimes resolve long-standing conflicts if each partner accepts and understands the differences in each other's perceptions and can use that knowledge to better support one another in later conflicts. Often just learning that a word or sentence has a totally different meaning for each of you can be a key to resolving hurt feelings. The best kind of validation you can give is to offer understanding to your partner. Note that this doesn't mean you have to believe your partner was 100 percent correct in their assessment of what happened. This also doesn't mean that you have to capitulate and start defining yourself and your actions wholly based on your partner's perception. You each have your own reality, and nobody has a monopoly on what is true, so it can be restorative to hear something like, "I can see how that would be really scary to feel like you were being abandoned."

After one person shares their experience, trade roles so the second person becomes the one sharing and the first person is now the listener.

H IS FOR HISTORY

While the first step is about learning how each of you experienced this particular conflict or fight, the second step is about sharing how the fight and the emotions it generated relate to your past. Most emotions that get activated during conflict aren't new or unfamiliar. So much of our emotional response is recycled pain dredged up to the surface by someone brushing up against our tender spots. For this step you will again take turns sharing and listening. The speaker will share any connections that the fight or emotions had to their past pain, while the listener uses their best listening skills to learn more about their partner and how their experiences might affect the way they relate to one another.

If you are the partner sharing, this is where you will work to find connections between this quarrel and any enduring vulner-abilities or triggers that occurred in the past—especially ones from before the current relationship began. You may have already gotten some insights into these connections while sharing your story in step one. If not, this step is where you can search your memory for points in your history when you had a similar set of feelings. If you can identify any of these moments, take time to share this with your partner so they can understand why this particular event may have had extra emotional weight for you. This could range from mild frustrations to triggers from child-hood experiences, pain from a previous breakup, accumulated wounds from being a member of a marginalized group, exposure to frightening or violent events, or any other past trauma.

In addition to connecting your feelings to past experiences, this is also a chance to clarify any beliefs you may have about the meaning of certain actions or words. For example, a person may believe that punctuality is a sign of consideration and that being late means you are uncaring. These types of beliefs are often deeply rooted in us from childhood, sometimes from being taught explicitly by our families, but most often through the examples that our caregivers set while we were growing up. These beliefs may never change, so the purpose of this exercise is not to unlearn them but to aim for understanding each other's beliefs while showing each other that you care.

As the listener, your job is to hear your partner out with empathy, compassion, and understanding. Being a good listener doesn't mean sitting silently; it can also include clarifying questions or acknowledgments. Again, make an effort to keep your focus on listening and understanding, rather than correcting your partner or inserting your own opinions. Absolutely do *not* try to tell them why their belief is wrong or try to convince them not to feel a certain way. Not only will those tactics be ineffective, but it is likely to derail and shut down the entire effort to repair and reconnect. They may adjust their beliefs over time, but not because you logic-ed them into it during a discussion. Remember: your partner is someone you love because of who *they* are, not because they're a mirror image of you and your beliefs.

After one person has finished sharing about their history, we highly encourage offering some empathy and validation before switching roles. Even something as simple as "I understand a little better why you would feel the way you did" goes a long, long way toward lowering defenses and helping your partner feel seen and heard.

O IS FOR OWNERSHIP

After both people have shared their story of what happened in the fight and have explored how feelings and reactions may be related to personal histories, you should begin to have a better understanding of why the conflict materialized and escalated in the first place. The next step in our repair process is about exploring which parts of the fight you can take ownership of. Remember, you both care about each other, and most likely neither one of you was maliciously trying to hurt the other. In most arguments, there are certain things each of you can take responsibility for. If you truly believe that your partner was intentionally hurting you, and if these infringements have been occurring over an extended period of time, then we recommend you read the It's Okay to Break Up section in Extra Tools.

Ownership may mean you acknowledge one or several things you could have done better during the disagreement. It could be accepting that you made a major mistake or simply owning up to a small contribution to the argument. In any case, this step is extremely beneficial to repairing the relationship. Research from the Gottman Institute has found that even taking responsibility for a single, small part of the communication breakdown can offer an opportunity for repair.

Evita "Lavitaloca" Sawyers, creator of *Today's Polyamory Reminder*, makes an apt observation: "Learning to differentiate between what our feelings are, what our needs are, and what our observations and judgments are is a huge aid to helping us determine what is ours and what is someone else's shit.

"So, 'I lashed out at you because I was angry that you stayed out all night with your other partner and didn't text me to let me know you were okay or not coming back home. You're so inconsiderate!' becomes 'You stayed out all night with your other partner and didn't text me to let me know you were safe and not coming home. I was worried about you and hurt, because I thought that you didn't think about me during your evening to tell me that you weren't coming home. I spoke harshly to you, because while I needed to express my pain and anger, I was too emotional at the time to do so calmly.'

"Understanding that people aren't to blame for our feelings or what behaviors we choose in response to those feelings helps with our own awareness of what our contribution is to whatever conflict we may be experiencing with a person."

Owning up to mistakes, especially if the behavior felt valid at the time, can be especially difficult if you come from a culture or family where admitting any fault is equivalent to losing an argument. If you realize that taking ownership is a struggle for you, you can begin by admitting that fact to your partner. Recognizing and stating out loud that it is a challenge for you is a good point of entry. With practice and support from your partner, the owner-ship step will become easier over time. If you've tried everything, but this step is still challenging for you, take a look at the trouble-shooting section later in this chapter for more tips. Sawyers also offers advice on this: "I think of what I would want my partners to do for me if the tables were turned. I would want them to hold themselves accountable. I would want them to be self-aware. I would want them to take ownership of their humanity. So that's what I do."

P IS FOR PREVENTION

After sharing and understanding each other's stories of what happened during the fight, exploring how your histories are connected to that experience, and taking ownership of your part in the conflict, it can be tempting to pat yourselves on the back and call it a day. You've done some amazing work up to this point, and you probably have a much better understanding of each other's inner worlds and are equipped to be more empathetic moving forward. However, the final step, prevention, is what takes you that extra mile from just understanding why a fight occurred to preventing it from escalating again in the future.

In the prevention step, you will discuss together how you might do things differently next time a similar conflict comes up. Ask each other, "What is one thing that we each can do to stop an annoyance or disagreement from growing into a full-on fight? What is one thing that I will try to do differently, and what's one thing that my partner could do differently?" Even after going through the previous steps, it is still easy to follow old neural pathways and habits that lead to similar conflict. From the time we were children, through years of conditioning, we carve certain mental grooves that can be easy to slip into and difficult to get out of. These are the patterns that cause us to respond poorly to something by swearing, slamming doors, using the silent treatment, or doing other hurtful and unproductive behavior. To combat this, it can be helpful to think of positive methods or behaviors that you use to fight a bad habit. We all have patterns of behavior that are less than ideal, but we also have the power to start changing them.

As we've discussed before, trying to consciously change your behavior while you are emotionally activated is extremely difficult. That is why the prevention step is so important. It gives us a chance to prepare and plan ahead when we are in an unemotional state so that we don't have to come up with solutions in the moment when it's too late. These habitual patterns and neural pathways are also easier to change the earlier you notice them and course correct. An example of habitual patterns in conflict are what we call Demon Dance Battles, which you can learn more about in the Extra Tools section.

Microscripts (see Chapter 4) are one of our favorite ways to avoid going down the same negative path the next time conflict arises. A Microscript works well because it's planned in advance, so it has a connection to a time when you were calmer and more compassionate. As a bonus, it's extremely easy to use: you just say your specific script. Yes, it can feel awkward and silly, but sometimes that little taste of fun is enough to help break the negative pattern.

The key to this step is for the two of you to work together to come up with ways for both of you to defuse a situation and minimize hurt feelings in the future. You can still disagree, and you may still be hurt, but this preventative step can avoid the unproductive blowups that cause damage and rarely resolve anything.

THE SECRET BONUS STEP: RECONNECT

For our extra-credit students out there, there's a bonus step that we like to tack on at the end of this process—reconnect. This involves you and your partner intentionally coming back to a state of appreciation and connection through offering compliments, expressing gratitude, rewarding yourselves with a favorite treat, or sharing some loving touch. This step isn't mandatory. Even though the repair process may have gone smoothly, one or both partners may feel better taking some space from one another or engaging in a pleasant distraction before coming back together. However, if you have the bandwidth and time to reconnect, we encourage you to do so. If not, you can still congratulate yourselves on getting through a repair process. As an extra-special bonus, you get to add an R to the end of the acronym, and you can say you are a secret SHOPR! (Do secret shoppers still exist?) We'll talk much more about the power of reconnection in Chapter 7.

The Most Common Relationship Issues

There are hundreds of experiences, personality differences, and variations in values that can cause couples to fight. Many of those situations are unique to the couple experiencing them. However, despite the idiosyncrasies of each relationship, the most common issues tend to fall into the same few categories. Repair SHOP was created to help couples mend their relationships no matter what type of issue they are facing. Ideally, if you build an awareness of the patterns you and your partner tend to cycle through, you can learn to have a proactive mind-set, more effectively defuse an argument while it is happening, or repair the relationship after a fight has occurred. Even those "perpetual problems" that never seem to get fully resolved can be more easily dealt with by using our Repair SHOP method. So, what are some of the most common relationship disagreements people tend to go through, and how can the Repair SHOP help them?

MISCOMMUNICATION
No one out there can communicate effectively 100 percent of the time. While the tools in this book are designed to aid in communication issues, it is still possible to say something we don't really mean, communicate in a confusing way, or have a communication style that is simply different from our partner's. Just as it takes years to truly understand another person, it can take years to learn how to effectively communicate with a partner. Miscommunication can also include a lack of understanding of what each of you wants out of the relationship. One partner may want a traditional relationship-escalator style of commitment, while the other is more interested in a nonhierarchical type of entanglement. Whatever the reason, communicating at cross-purposes can cause many frustrating arguments.

The story step of SHOP is especially helpful in this type of argument. The story step is all about listening, and often misunderstandings can occur when two people aren't really hearing one another. After listening to your partner's story about what they just felt and observed during the argument, ask clarifying questions to help better your understanding of how they viewed the issue. Each of you should give time and space for the other to fully discuss their viewpoint and then take turns asking questions without falling into the trap of dismissal or defensiveness.

MONEY

Many experts and researchers have found that money and financial problems are a leading cause of divorce in the United States. Most of us are socialized to have complicated feelings surrounding money, and those feelings and habits may extend to how we view finances in a relationship. How each partner chooses to spend their money, substantial differences in what each partner makes, and how each person financially contributes to the relationship are just some of the ways in which money can cause anxiety and anger to bubble up and spill over.

When we aim to get a clearer understanding about what money means to our partner, it is important to recognize where their habits and viewpoints around money came from. Enter the history step. When you reach this part of Repair SHOP, get curious. Ask if there are specific beliefs instilled from your partner's family of origin that may have contributed to disagreements around money. Recognize if those beliefs are vastly different from your own. Question whether either of you has a pattern of using words or phrases around money that are unintentionally upsetting. Learning about your partner's past can provide important information, especially when each of you has different viewpoints on how to handle and spend your money. With this information, you can both begin working toward creating a plan for how money can be a beneficial tool in your relationship, not a cringe-worthy conversation to avoid.

FAMILY

The old adage says to never discuss sex, money, or family on a first date. While the common trope of "the unbearable in-laws" may feel dated, it's true that you can't pick your family or the family of your significant other. A partner's family member might not approve of your relationship, express bigoted or unkind sentiments around you, or generally just be a pain in the ass to be around. There are a whole host of other challenges that family can present, and this is especially relevant in some cases if your relationship does not fall on the traditional, heteronormative spectrum. So when it comes to fights about family, how do you avoid your discussions devolving into resentment, defensiveness, and chaos?

Our previous chapter on boundaries can offer key insights on how to protect yourself from any toxic people peripherally or intimately connected to your life. As difficult as it may be, deciding to cut or drastically reduce time spent with toxic people, including family members, is the prerogative of you and your significant other. When each of you don't agree on those shared boundaries, it is possible for arguments to arise. This is an area where the prevention step can come into play. All of the other SHOP steps can also be helpful when discussing family, but prevention can help both of you compromise and work together to make sure you each feel comfortable and cared for in the presence of each other's families. Get creative with your partner and make a plan of action for the next time family comes into town. Decide on a way to bail out if one or both of you feels like it's time to take a break from the visit. Use Microscripts to let each other know it's okay in the moment if something a family member says is triggering. The prevention step can bring you both together so that you each feel understood, cared for, and part of each other's team the next time a family-related grievance occurs.

CHORES AND LABOR

We are all familiar with the traditional heteronormative view of relationships where men make the money and women take care of the home. These gender roles persisted for decades and have only started to truly evolve and change in the last few decades. Today, the modern couple strives to have a much more egalitarian division of labor when it comes to monetary contributions to the household, child rearing, and household chores. Yet deeply ingrained social norms, lessons from our families of origin, and differing beliefs in how tidy a household should be kept can still cause tremendous conflict between cohabiting partners.

This is another area where the history and prevention steps can be extremely beneficial by providing insight about the kinds of things a partner was taught in their youth regarding household labor, and then creating an action plan for both partners to use when rebalancing the division of labor. An additional, vital step that can be useful during this type of argument is the ownership step. Ownership is not only about taking credit for the parts of the argument that you could have handled better, but also owning how much (or how little) household labor you actually partake in. An American Family Survey found that men think they have an even fifty-fifty split when it comes to dividing household labor with their female partners. However, the majority of studies and surveys posit the bulk of household labor disproportionately falls on women, especially when children are involved.

Owning the reality of how much labor you or your partner does is the first step toward creating a more equal partnership. Chores are not only about tidying up the house; they also include the mental load of planning, organizing, and decision-making. Recognizing and owning the differences between two partners' mental loads is important to consider when collaborating during

197

the prevention step. Deeply ingrained beliefs are hard to change, yet taking ownership can help couples move in a direction of equality and prosperity for the relationship.

VALUES

What do we want out of life? How do we choose to live our life on a daily basis? What are our goals and what is our ultimate purpose? The answers to these questions are personal and will often align with the people with whom you choose to have relationships. However, when two people's core values are misaligned, conflict can arise easily. Decisions like whether or not to have children, whether or not to cohabitate, differences in where you each want the relationship to go, and if you want to be monogamous or poly-amorous can put even the healthiest of relationships at a crossroad (if you are unsure of what your values are, we recommend our exercise on finding your values in the Extra Tools section).

Values are ideally something that should be discussed early in a relationship, but there is always a potential that one partner will try to align with another partner's values, only to find that ulti-mately their expectations are let down. As personal and profound as values are, a misalignment doesn't necessarily spell relation-ship doom. This is where history and prevention can help part-ners learn more about each other's backstory and see if they can compromise and move in a direction that satisfies parts of both of their values. Perhaps one partner grew up in a highly tradi-tional household and has had a lifelong dream of having a family and getting married. Another partner might want to break free of the constraints they felt while growing up and seek nonnormative connections. While values can be altered throughout the course of one's life, it is important to try to not change your partner's values in hopes they may become more aligned with your own.

The prevention step can be a great tool for discussing and

coming up with ideas for how you can stay entangled even if you want different things. You may decide that de-escalating the relationship or transitioning it into a friendship is the best solution for the both of you. Transitions can be challenging, but as we always say on the show (as well as in the Extra Tools section), it's okay to break up. A difference in values doesn't mean you have to leave each other, and SHOP can help you each make an informed decision on the overall quality of your relationship even if you ultimately are looking for different things.

IRRECONCILABLE DIFFERENCES

Loss of trust. Lack of sexual intimacy. Political differences. Substance abuse. Addiction. *Irreconcilable differences* is the catchall term for the issues that couples simply cannot come to terms with. These often fall under the umbrella of those "perpetual" problems that we discussed earlier in this chapter (especially when they become "gridlocked" problems. More on that later in the chapter). How do two people deal with the irreconcilable differences that plague their relationship? Is it even possible to have a healthy relationship with persistent issues present?

Truly, it depends on the severity of the issue and the frequency with which it is causing strife in the relationship. With concerns like substance abuse and addiction, a course of action using the prevention step is an important first tactic for each of you to begin making a plan for possible rehabilitation. Twelve-step programs, rehabilitation centers, and specialized therapy are some of the many ways to seek help for substance abuse. It may be time to ask yourselves if these issues are deal breakers for your relationship.

When it comes to issues that are not as potentially life altering, the couple must question if they feel like the relationship could continue even if the issue was never resolved. As we discussed earlier, many perpetual problems, while challenging, are simply differences that couples learn to live with over time. In fact, the Gottman Institute's research says that only around 31 percent of issues are solvable! While this seems like a grim number, it goes to show that many couples can thrive even if they still have some perpetual issues that plague their day-to-day lives.

So how can we deal with irreconcilable, unsolvable differences? Every element of Repair SHOP should be utilized in these scenarios. First, identify each other's stories surrounding the problem. Discuss exactly how it makes each of you feel when the problem occurs, as well as any patterns of emotional responses that persistently flare up. Second, talk about your history surrounding the issue. Maybe you grew up in a family where punctuality was a necessary trait, and you would be punished for being late. Perhaps you feel like your partner is disrespecting you when they are late. Next, take ownership of your part of the problem. Yes, your partner may not be on time, but the issue spins out of control when you have a habit of rolling your eyes and shaking your head every time they are late. Lastly, figure out a plan of action with the prevention step. Maybe your partner will endeavor to come ten minutes early to every engagement the two of you have this month. Maybe you can endeavor to graciously smile and appreciate their efforts, regardless of whether or not they happen to achieve timeliness. If the two of you already know of a perpetual problem, you don't even need to have an argument about it before implementing these steps. Take an hour on a weekend to talk about the issue and work through the Repair SHOP steps with your partner. Or better yet, schedule a RADAR session where you can create a dedicated space to air grievances, talk about future plans and goals with your partner, and get each other up to speed on the comings and goings of each other's lives. We will discuss all things RADAR in the next chapter.

Lyla and Kevin's Repair SHOP

This is how Lyla and Kevin used the Repair SHOP steps to process their argument:

STORY

Kevin began by laying out the story from his perspective: "I was having a pretty good evening to myself, but then I looked at the clock and noticed that it was already a half hour past when you told me you'd get back home. At first, I didn't think too much of it, but as it got later, I started feeling upset. I felt worried that maybe you'd gotten in an accident, and then I felt annoyed and angry that you might have just forgotten about me. I got a text from you around midnight, and then you arrived back at home about ten minutes later. I heard you walk in the door, and I was expecting you to apologize for being late. You walked into the kitchen and didn't say anything, so I asked what happened that caused you to be so late. You started explaining why you were late." He continued on with his version of events, finally concluding with, "And by that point, I was just too tired to keep arguing, so I fell asleep."

For Lyla, it was difficult at times to suppress the urge to interject or correct Kevin on his telling of the story, but she did her best to sit quietly and listen with compassion. Once he was finished, she took her turn.

"I was out at the bar with Sarah, and we were just about to head out the door when we were surprised by her brother walking in. Sarah has been talking to me for weeks about how excited she is for me to meet her family, so I decided to stay a little longer to introduce myself. I was trying hard to be present and make a good impression, and I forgot to text you about the change in plans. I didn't remember our agreement until I was already on the way home, which is when I texted you.

"When I walked into the room, I saw that your shoulders were tense and that you weren't smiling. I felt anxious, so I walked into the kitchen to give you a little space first. You asked me why I was late. I started explaining the situation, and before I could finish, you said that I was self-centered."

Lyla felt old feelings of hurt welling up in her chest. She paused for a moment and took a slow breath before continuing to the end of her story. "I worried that we were just going to keep talking around each other, and I knew that if I forced myself to stay awake, it would just get worse. So I told you that I couldn't talk about this anymore, and I got into bed."

Kevin also did his best to hold steady and listen to Lyla's version of the story. Both of them had slightly different versions of the events, and each person had different moments that stood out in their memory. For each of them, hearing these differences was sometimes challenging but also offered compelling insight into what was going on in each other's inner worlds. Once both had taken their turns, they agreed to move on to the next step.

HISTORY

Kevin sat for a few minutes to gather his thoughts before sharing. "This incident set off some of my own painful baggage from the past. I know I've already told you about how my dad would sometimes completely space out picking me up from school. It feels a little silly to bring that into this discussion, but I felt a similar mix of loneliness and rage coming up inside me. Because of that, I was in a pretty bad headspace by the time that you got home. On top of the anger, I had also been freaked out by the idea that something bad might have happened to you. I was so upset that I didn't care what excuse you might have had."

Lyla nodded slowly. "I remember when you shared that story about your dad with me. I know that's something that you've struggled with healing, and it makes sense why this situation would bring you right back into that again." Kevin also nodded, some tears welling up. Lyla continued on, sharing her history.

"It was really hard for me to hear you say I was self-centered. Once I heard those words, I completely lost it and didn't want to hear anything else you had to say. I knew inside that it was understandable to be upset, but all I could feel was that pain. 'Self-centered' was a descriptor that my ex would unfairly use against me all the time. It just brought me right back to that time. Also, I was excited and anxious to finally meet Sarah's brother. I wanted so badly to make a good first impression, and in the moment, I just got so focused on not blowing it that nothing else was on my mind."

Kevin felt a twinge of guilt. "I just assumed your date with Sarah was just a regular date," he said. "But now that I know the stakes were suddenly higher for you, it makes a lot more sense."

OWNERSHIP

The two had come to the next stage: taking ownership. They had done an excellent job of listening without interrupting, as well as offering validation of each other's experiences. They both hesitated at the ownership step. Feelings were still a little bit raw, and the idea of jumping straight into apologies was daunting. Despite this, Kevin began. "I can take responsibility for the fact that I didn't listen to you. I started from the beginning with the assumption that you didn't care at all, which wasn't fair of me. Also, I shouldn't have interrupted you, or accused you of being self-centered." He paused before adding, "I'm sorry for that."

Lyla took in a breath and said, "I appreciate that," before continuing. "It was harsh of me to tell you that this wasn't a big deal. That was pretty dismissive of your feelings. I do regret that I didn't text you earlier. I could have been more aware of the time."

And that was all for their ownership step. It wasn't long or drawn-out. There was no extensive self-castigating. It was simple yet poignant for both of them.

PREVENTION
Now it was time to get down to brass tacks. How could they avoid running into this pitfall in the future?

"I really don't mind if something comes up that means you'll be late. Even if plans totally change and you decide to stay the night somewhere else, that's fine by me," Kevin offered. "I can probably be more flexible about changing plans, but the most important thing for me is being kept in the loop and knowing what to expect."

"Yeah, I know. I'm the same way," Lyla said. "I do have a habit of spacing out on time, though. What if I tried setting an alarm on my phone for an hour before I told you I'd be home? That can be my reminder to update you on whether or not my plans have changed. Would that work?"

"That sounds like a good experiment to start with," Kevin said.

"I'd also like it to be okay for one of us to ask to table a discussion if it's getting too late at night," Lyla said. "Neither of us are at our best right before bed, and this isn't the first time that a conversation has spiraled late at night. Can we agree that it's okay to ask for a pause and pick up a conversation the next morning?"

Kevin nodded. "Yeah, we should be better about that. Let's give it a try."

Though it wasn't easy, Kevin and Lyla managed to get through the Repair SHOP process and came out the other side with a little more understanding, a little more empathy, and a little more ease transitioning back into their loving connection. That's the fundamental goal of repair: carefully paving a better pathway forward that pivots away from allowing the same conflict to happen again in the future.

Troubleshooting Your Repair SHOP

So you've learned all about the Repair SHOP, maybe thought about a few past arguments, and practiced some scenarios in your head where the SHOP steps could be utilized with your partner. Then an argument with your partner happens and . . . crap! Your Repair SHOP isn't working out like you planned! For those extra-tricky contingencies that seem to make your Repair SHOP especially challenging, we've outlined a few helpful ways to trouble-shoot your attempts to make amends.

WHEN WE START TO GO THROUGH THE REPAIR SHOP STEPS, WE GET PULLED BACK INTO THE FIGHT.

You and your partner have just reached the conclusion of a fight. You've read about Repair SHOP, want to reconnect, and have the best intentions for mending hurt and misunderstanding. You start discussing your stories and—wham! You find yourselves pulled back into the initial fight. Wait, what went wrong?

Emotions tend to run high during and directly after an argument. The term *flooding* refers to the release of hormones by your amygdala that readies the body for fight or flight. When we get into an argument with our partner, we (hopefully!) aren't also going to have to evade the attacks of a bear; however, the body's response readies you for just that. It's why we can relate to terms like *seeing red* and *losing your cool*: because the body is getting ready for action by creating a huge hormone-based emotional response.

How can you tell if you're getting into flooding territory? The physiological indicators of flooding are increased adrenaline, raised blood pressure, elevated pulse, and an activated sympathetic nervous system. Of all those, the easiest one to check is your pulse. If your pulse is over one hundred beats per minute, you are in floodtown, meaning you are physically incapable of listening and taking in what your partner is saying. If that is the case, stop and take some time for your body to regulate itself.

Researchers have found that it takes around twenty minutes for flooding hormones to leave the body. With that in mind, it may be helpful to call a time-out or HALT (more in the Extra Tools section) to allow both of you to calm down after a fight. Try not to exacerbate your feelings by venting to another person about what just occurred. Instead, do something relaxing to take your mind off the fight. This can include retreating into separate rooms, going on a short walk, meditating, playing video games, or reading a book to relieve yourself of anxiety and tension. After you feel like your body and brain are sufficiently calm, return to one another and try working through the SHOP steps.

There are times when a short HALT won't necessarily do the trick, however. If the fight between you and your partner was particularly nasty, included name-calling and shouting, or caused one or both of you to have an extreme emotional response, you may need to take a day or two for that emotional hurt to begin to dissipate. When both of you are ready, try coming back to the problem with a desire to understand your partner, to mend any hurt you may have caused during the argument, and to create a plan of action for the next time the issue occurs.

I don't know how to talk to my partner about my history.
Sharing past baggage and traumatic early experiences can be difficult for even the most open of individuals. Sometimes it's challenging to even know where to begin. And when you finally do

recall a painful memory and recognize that it may be influencing your current relationship, you might not know how to best tell your partner about it without getting defensive. Author and sex educator Tristan Taormino explains it like this: "Being able to open up emotionally to another person can be both exhilarating and terrifying. When we bring our whole selves to a relationship, that means everything, including past experiences, wounds, trauma. Many of us wear a certain amount of armor to protect ourselves from being hurt."

Taormino also shares her advice for having these discussions: "Talk to a partner or friend about what holds you back from allowing yourself to feel vulnerable. Naming the fear can help soften its hold on you. Be gentle with yourself and take your time. Sometimes you have to take the leap to expose your tender spots to someone."

To begin the process of having honest and vulnerable conversations around challenging subjects, here are some example sentences you can use as a starting point for sharing your history in a healthy, productive, and kind way:

- *"I need to talk to you about something that happened with my father when I was a kid, because I think it relates to how prickly I get when you ask me to do chores early in the morning. Can we try saving chore conversations for midday or the afternoon?"*

- *"I know that this isn't something that you are trying to do, but when I'm interrupted, I'm reminded of how I felt at my last job. I was usually the only nonwhite person at every meeting, and it felt like everyone had free license to talk over me*

> or talk down to me. It just brings me right back
> there."

- "We haven't really talked about this before, but money is a challenging subject for me. My parents were stressed about their money when I was growing up, and it caused me to be anxious about it as well. When I hear how much you want to go out to expensive places on dates, it makes me a little nervous that I won't be able to afford other expenses."

- "I know it's weird, but when I was growing up, the only compliments my grandfather ever gave me were about my appearance. My other siblings were told how smart and impressive they were, but I was just told how attractive I was. I appreciate that you find me sexy, but maybe you can try to focus your compliments on other aspects that you love about me for the next couple of months?"

- "I apologize for bracing myself and getting overly anxious every time we get into a little tiff. Whenever I would point something out to my ex, they would get defensive and start yelling at me. I think I have some baggage around arguments, even if they are fairly minor."

Hopefully some of these examples can get the wheels turning and help you feel more empowered and confident the next time you discuss your history with your partner. If you find yourself going through a chronic emotional pattern and are struggling to figure out where it is coming from, it might be helpful to try to remember the first time you felt that intense emotion. This may help you pinpoint the moment when the traumatic incident originated. When recalling past baggage, especially any trauma that has caused PTSD, we recommend speaking to a therapist to make sure you are getting the help you need when working through particularly painful memories.

I hate losing a fight! I always feel like I need to win!!
If you Google the words *win a fight*, not only will you be presented with a cascade of wikiHow articles on street fight tactics and videos of ripped dudes telling you the best way to drop an opponent, but you will also get served up psychological how-tos and sneaky tactics on "Basic Training for Verbal Combat." While this all sounds like a lot of fun, it definitely is NOT how you want to go about defusing or even having an argument with the person you are in a relationship with. This is a sticking point that is near and not so dear for Dedeker.

DEDEKER SAYS

"Conflict resolution" was a foreign concept in the household I grew up in. There's been a long family tradition of authoritarianism, which meant that in any conflict, you fight and fight and fight until there is a clear winner and a clear loser. If you're the winner, that means that you were loud enough and angry enough to get the last word. If you're the loser, that means you're at fault, and you had better shape up before you expect any kindness or sense of resolution. There were no examples of apologizing or taking respon-

---

sibility for raised voices or harsh words spoken in the heat of anger. I rocketed into my adult relationships in this way, believing that the only way to have healthy conflict was to either assure that you could win or to not have conflict at all.

Depending on your situation growing up, you may have been privy to watching the people who raised you do anything from shouting and slamming doors to passive-aggressive eye-rolling and flat out ignoring each other. Many of us don't have a good model for how to fight *well* and have next to no standards on how to make up in a healthy way. If the adults in our life did reconnect and repair after a fight, that part may have happened privately, behind closed doors, even if the blowup occurred publicly in the kitchen. And for some of us, admitting any wrongdoing feels like we are admitting to being a failure. We want to *win* the fight, have the last word, and make the other person know how much they screwed up and how right *we* were.

The problem is this generally gets us nowhere and can ultimately lead to a slew of problems for our relationships in the future. So if you are reading this and deep down you know this is something you do, try to pause and take a breath the next time you have the urge to say the last word and win the fight. Instead, try to recognize what you did wrong in the fight, take responsibility, and tell your partner you will do better next time. Remember that even taking ownership of one small part of the problem can still be effective. Our partners are not our enemies, and ideally it should be the two of you against the problem, not the two of you against each other. So buck up, set aside your ego, and find a way to say you're sorry. That powerful word might get you both on a path to understanding, vulnerability, and renewed trust.

It's hard to not take everything my partner is telling me super personally.

Books, television, podcasts, and media all tell us that "the one" is out there, try to instruct us on how to nab the perfect mate, and imply that your self-worth should be predicated on whether or not you have a relationship. All that external chatter can place a lot of pressure and expectations on you and the person you fall in love with. That's why, when your partner is telling you something about you that they have an issue with, it can feel like such an intense and devastating blow! *How could this person think this about me? Do they even know who I am? I feel like they're telling me I'm a terrible partner!*

As hard as it may sound, stepping back and looking at the big picture is an important skill to learn in moments like this. The ability to see a situation from thirty thousand feet can be vital when hearing that your partner has a problem with something in your relationship. First of all, get curious about both your history and the history of your partner. When the two of you reach the second step of Repair SHOP, commit to actively listen to the things they are telling you! Did something in their past cause them to react to what you did in a certain way? Is something that feels insignificant to you a big problem to them because they were raised a particular way? Was there something about your own behavior or misstep in the past that influenced their perception of your communication today?

As partners, it is important to be gentle around each other's emotional triggers. Ideally, the most empathetic and caring of couples will learn how to pick up the slack when one of them is having a difficult time, understand that an issue might be a *them* problem and not a *you* problem, and try to adjust a behavior so their partner feels validated and cared for. We all have loads of challenging experiences in our past that shape who we are today and how we operate in our daily lives. The next time your partner says you are doing something that annoys or hurts them, instead of getting defensive, step back, look at the bigger picture, and ask yourself if it's really about you or them.

This thing that the two of us are fighting about never seems to get resolved, no matter what we do.

As we mentioned earlier, 69 percent of recurring arguments come from perpetual, fundamental differences between two people that are not ever going to be resolved. A big example that has come up often in our lives is dating a person who ultimately wants a monogamous relationship while we were more interested in a polyamorous one. While many couples make mono/polyam relationships work, others find the difference in lifestyle needs are simply not compatible and choose to end the relationship, or make some drastic compromises. What counts as a perpetual problem can be different from couple to couple. One couple might call something a perpetual problem while another couple might see it as simply a difference of opinion that two people can learn to live with.

Sometimes, perpetual problems can turn into what the Gottmans call a "gridlocked problem." These are issues that have been poorly handled by the couple over a period of time and now feel unsafe to bring up or discuss. The issue feels gridlocked, at a painful standstill, and neither of you feels any positive movement when it happens to rear its ugly head. Some partners understand that a perpetual problem may never be resolved, and that is totally okay with them. A partner may just always be untidy, and even if it's not ideal, the other person recognizes this as a playful idiosyncrasy or a difference in lifestyle choice. However, if that same problem is met with anger, frustration, and disappointment over and over again, it can cause the issue to become gridlocked. One person may feel shame at being unable to change. The other person may feel like their partner doesn't care about them and their needs. These problems can spiral out of control, lead to both people being overcritical of one another when the issue arises, and, over a long period of time, ultimately spell doom for the relationship.

Learning to strengthen your communication skills, working to see your partner as a team member and not the enemy, and being curious about your partner's past history can all help end the cycle of the gridlocked problem. There are underlying reasons for any relationship problem or personality trait that cause partners to be at odds with one another. You have to be willing to dig deep, ask questions, listen hard, and try to understand your partner's intentions, pains, hopes, and dreams. Once you can begin to do these things, you can begin to fully appreciate your partners for who they are, regardless of their personality traits or eccentricities. And again, it can be helpful to get a professional involved to help you and your partner get to the bottom of these sorts of issues.

Homework

To begin applying Repair SHOP in your relationships, it's imperative to get the other person onboard. Start by reading this chapter together with your partner, and talk about what emotions it brings up. You or your partner may see the steps as an obvious way to aid in repair, or you may see the method as theoretical, rigid, or awkward. In either case, absorbing the information and having a conversation about how to best utilize the steps in your relationship can be a helpful starting point. If you read this chapter early in a relationship, before you've even had any fights, great! You'll be better equipped to handle fights in healthier ways when they come and can quickly work on repairing them before they become any more toxic.

If you are unsure or apprehensive about beginning the repair process, go easy on yourself. Together with your partner, try to think of a past argument or disagreement that was relatively low stakes. It will be easier the less emotional charge there is for both of you. You could pick an older disagreement that hasn't been a repeated fight just to try out the tool and see how it feels, or you could even pick something slightly silly and inconsequential just to get used to the steps. Even with a small disagreement, you may be surprised to learn how each of your perceptions of what happened are slightly different. If you're lucky, you may even gain some important insights into each other's pasts. The goal of this homework is to practice the steps before you need to apply them in a more difficult situation.

And lastly, go back to your homework from Chapter 1. What are you longing for here? What would the ability to repair past conflict mean for your relationship?

Repair SHOP Cheat Sheet

Like so many of the tools we have spent hours discussing on the *Multiamory* podcast, Repair SHOP was created to help people stop being *reactive* and start being *proactive* about their relationship disagreements. Though it might be challenging in the heat of the moment, couples who practice Repair SHOP on a regular basis can use the SHOP steps to prevent arguments from escalating into blowup fights. To recap, here are all of the Repair SHOP steps again, as well as some questions to ask yourselves the next time you and your partner are in the aftermath of an argument. Remember to take turns speaking and listening at each step.

1. **Stories**—How did each of you interpret the disagreement that just occurred? Tell each other your story of what happened. Listen closely and see how your story might be different from your partner's story.

2. History—Do you have any triggers that might have caused you to feel challenged by something your partner said or did? Do you have a core belief that acted as a catalyst for the argument? Relay your history to your partner and/or ask if something in their history caused them to feel pain around this issue.

3. Ownership—It takes two to tango. Ask yourself what you could have done better during the argument. Accept responsibility for your actions and for the parts of the fight that you contributed to. Apologize if it's appropriate.

4. Prevention—How can we make it better next time? What did we learn from this fight? What is one thing that I could do differently, and what is one thing my partner could do differently? Create a plan together with your partner on how you both can do better next time.

Takeaways

- A lack of repair attempts in a relationship can lead to a buildup of resentment, a decrease in vulner-ability/authenticity, as well as a rise in negativity between partners.

- Sixty-nine percent of all conflicts are perpetual, unsolvable problems. Relationships start to flounder when these perpetual problems become "gridlocked."

- It probably isn't possible to find a partner who is 100 percent compatible with you, so . . .

- Use the Repair SHOP steps to help repair conflict, whether it's perpetual or not!

  > Stories
  > History
  > Ownership
  > Prevention

- Give yourself time and space away from a fight before you attempt the Repair SHOP steps. Make sure you are in a steady place physiologically.

- Take *ownership* and responsibility for your actions in conflict.

- Try not to take your partner's feedback so personally! Sometimes an issue your partner has is related to their *story* of what happened during a fight and their past *history*.

- Work with your partner in a kind and empathetic way to ensure you can *prevent* similar conflict in the future. As an extra bonus, take the time to *reconnect*.

For more information, check out *Multiamory* Episode 234, "SHOP: How to Repair after a Fight."

CHAPTER 7

RADAR:
Effective Relationship Check-Ins

P hil and Oscar had reached a big snag in their relationship. After three years, their lust-filled, fiery, and exciting connection had begun to cool off, and conflict had become commonplace. They both still loved and cared deeply about each other, but their disagreements seemed to pop up at the worst times, and they did not know how to come to easy resolutions.

As much as he loved Oscar, Phil hated spending time with Oscar's family, especially Oscar's mother, who disliked their relationship and would occasionally make passive-aggressive comments about it. Oscar would usually say nothing instead of standing up to her and defending their partnership. Phil knew Oscar's mom was important to him, so for his sake, he would put on a brave face when they visited her. This felt like a noble sacrifice for the well-being of the relationship, and most of the time Phil was able to handle it. Yet, at seemingly random moments, he would get very upset, and a discussion about a totally different topic would turn into an argument about how Oscar didn't value their relationship enough to stand up to his mom. All those feelings of frustration would bubble up despite Phil's best efforts, and the conversation would leave Oscar surprised and confused as to what the argument was actually about. To make matters worse, this usually happened late in the evening, when both of them were tired, which meant the conversations were rarely productive.

Oscar had his own sore points, too. He was consistently upset over Phil's workaholic attitude and felt like their relationship was not a top priority to Phil. He knew that Phil took his work seriously, and when they first got together, it was a trait that he admired. Over time, however, it became harder to appreciate when he felt like his needs weren't being met. Oscar would be at his breaking point, most often during Phil's busiest times, when he had deadlines looming or needed to work in the evenings. This would lead Phil to look for a quick solution or to shut down the conversation so that he could finish his projects. He wanted to be there for Oscar and felt the best way to do so was to scramble to wrap up his work so they could spend time together. However, it was difficult to feel motivated to make bigger changes when Oscar would bring up grievances. To Oscar, it felt like Phil wasn't interested in fixing the issue of being overworked, and he would end up feeling even more hurt and neglected than before he brought it up.

Many of us will recognize the core underlying conflicts in Oscar and Phil's story, whether it's challenges about children, household chores, dating, quality time, or any number of other issues. In some relationships, there may be tension around certain subjects, and partners may question the timing of when to have a challenging discussion. Others may feel a constant struggle to find a balance between keeping one's mouth shut and toughing it out versus bringing up every little irritation as it happens. Whether you are seeking relief from a pattern of conflict, a way to unpack long-unresolved issues, a desire to rebuild trust, or just want to deepen an already solid connection, a regular relationship check-in may be your most effective tool. It was helpful for Phil and Oscar—more on that later.

Why have a relationship check-in at all?

It turns out that a regular relationship check-in is a surprisingly hard sell to most folks. *You want me to have . . . a meeting? About my relationship? Like . . . in a boardroom?* The image clashes with the usual picture we're served up about relationships: two people tangled up together in a pink cloud of romantic haze where no conflict dare enter, and they stay that way until the end of time. In reality, that haze gets cleared away pretty quickly when real-world problems arrive: unvoiced expectations, hurt feelings, schedule juggling, past trauma, differences in communication styles, and systemic challenges from within and without.

Having regular, intentional time set aside to care for and communicate about your relationship is paramount. The good news is that even if you have a regularly established relationship check-in, you can still talk about things organically as they come up. The addition of having a regular safe space for communication helps to bring up important topics before they turn into full-blown problems. This enables you to minimize day-to-day admin and processing while at the same time maximizing positive, nonprocessing time with your partner. It also prevents a problem backlog from building up until someone has to explode and unleash all their grievances at once. This is particularly important if you or your partner have a tendency toward conflict avoidance, which was a struggle for Lex and Rob.

Lex and Rob were the couple everyone else in their friend group looked up to. They were adorable together, loved hosting board game nights, and were both friendly and kind to one another. The fact that so many people admired them made Lex feel like even more of a failure when there were little things about the relationship that got under their skin. Lex was good at emotional regulation and almost never lost their cool. While Lex tried to accept there would always be some things that frustrated them, they were starting to worry that it was becoming harder to put on a happy face. Rob was caring and often went out of his way to do nice things for Lex, so they knew it wasn't anything he was doing on purpose, but there were small things he *didn't* do that would leave Lex feeling frustrated or upset. As an example, over the years Lex had mostly let Rob have the final say in how their apartment was decorated. He was a lot more passionate and vocal about his preferences, and Lex wanted him to be happy in their home, but he rarely asked about *Lex's* preferences for their place. If Rob did something unintentionally hurtful and Lex got upset, he would ask how to address the issue, but often Lex couldn't quite put their finger on why the behavior was upsetting. There was never a real opportunity to talk out their feelings with Rob. After the conflict dissipated, Lex was scared to bring it up again, worried that they would just be dredging up old hurts, something Lex knew Rob had hated about his last relationship.

Overall, Rob was happy in the relationship, too. He had small frustrations now and then, but they would get resolved as soon as he brought them up to Lex. The big thing weighing on Rob was the subtle ways in which he had seen Lex retreat inward over the years. When they had first gotten together, he loved Lex's zeal for life, their intelligence, and their outgoing personality. He couldn't quite identify how, but he had a feeling that some of that energy and their connection had diminished. He cared deeply about Lex and would sometimes try to bring it up, but Lex would usually react by apologizing and saying that they were just tired or give some other explanation. Even though they remained loving and kind toward one another, Rob worried that

Lex might be drifting away from him but had no idea what to do about it.

Rob and Lex prioritized avoiding conflict above all else, but this caused both of them to fail to learn how to communicate effectively with one another. Lex didn't want to rock the boat with Rob and therefore avoided airing grievances with him. Rob realized Lex was retreating inward but had no way to talk to them about it without stumbling into an uncomfortable confrontation.

Later on, we will circle back to this couple and explore how incorporating a RADAR helped to instill safety, confidence, and understanding into their communication. *What's RADAR?* Great question! In short, it is our framework for having safe, productive, and positive relationship check-ins. Before we get into the details of *what* it is, let's take some time to understand how it came to be and why it is important.

The History of RADAR

We created RADAR in 2017, but its history goes back to the eighties and nineties, when the agile methodology was first introduced to the business world. The revolutionary concept of agile scrum was created to move businesses away from large, fixed, linear project planning. Instead, agile methodologies embraced the idea that the best path forward may change on a daily basis. It altered the focus from large-scale goals to smaller, faster, more attainable goals, which could be reviewed and adjusted more often. Please don't fall asleep yet—it gets sexier, we promise.

In 2016, blogger Alanna Irving published a post called "Running Agile Scrum on Our Relationship," where she discussed how she and her partner took the agile scrum tools that they used every day in their work as software engineers and applied them to improving their relationship. As a result of having regular agile scrum check-ins, Irving reported that she and her partner were better able to divide household chores, grew more understanding of how to better support each other, and even made the decision to get married!

After reading the article, the three of us were intrigued but skeptical. Would this sort of framework really hold up over time? Would it work for people in less entwined relationships? What about couples who were intentionally not on the track toward marriage? What about relationships with more than two people? We decided to make ourselves the guinea pigs and committed to trying out the agile scrum framework in our own relationships for a year. After spending that year evaluating what worked, collecting feedback from listeners, and making changes, we released our own format for a regular monthly relationship check-in, and RADAR was born! The idea of taking a well-established business and planning process and adapting it for relationship maintenance was exciting (to us nerds, at least), but we found that a lot of people were put off by agile scrum because they already used it at work and felt it was too impersonal. When we developed RADAR, we intentionally focused on finding a balance between an objective methodology to help give structure to relationship discussions and the flexibility, intimacy, and uniqueness that make each relationship special.

After releasing our first episode about RADAR in 2017, we quickly began to realize we had stumbled on something special. More and more people began using it, recommended it to their friends and partners, and even brought it back full circle to use in their businesses. We have had therapists and counselors recommend it to their clients, educators teach workshops about it, and people around the world offer to translate it into other languages.

To this day, RADAR is one of our proudest creations because

of the sheer number of people it has helped by providing a structure to improve their relationship communication, address challenging topics in a safe way, and redirect the majority of their time to enjoying all the wonderful parts of their relationships.

The Research on Relationship Check-Ins

The three of us have seen firsthand how beneficial having a safe, scheduled, dedicated check-in time can be for a relationship. Ever since we debuted the RADAR model, hundreds of listeners have reached out to tell us how much RADAR has helped their relationships grow and thrive. You don't have to take our word for it, however, or even the word of our listeners. There is scientific evidence that regular check-ins can help sustain and enhance relationship health, much in the same way that a regular check-in with a doctor or therapist can support long-term physical and mental health.

The Marriage Checkup (MC), created by Clark University professor of psychology James V. Córdova, is a two-session checkup designed to evaluate and improve the health of a relationship. It was created to help married couples who were generally averse to seeking long-term couples' counseling improve their relationships in a shorter period of time. There are a lot of reasons for people to avoid seeking relationship counseling, including time, money, lack of childcare, and overall reluctance that therapy will help. A model like MC has been shown to work well, both for couples who are already having challenges in addition to those who simply want to be preventative when it comes to the health of their relationship.

The Marriage Checkup, much like our RADAR model, was designed to be less scary for couples interested in working through their relational issues. One 2014 study on the MC found that there was a 97 percent completion rate, and participants reported an overall increase in intimacy, acceptance, and satisfaction in their relationships. Couples reported still feeling this improvement even after six-month, one-year, and two-year follow-ups. The researchers came to the conclusion this kind of regular checkup served to care for long-term relationship health in a way that is more accessible (and more affordable) than long-term counseling.

We created RADAR in the same spirit. Working with a counselor or therapist can bring major benefits to your relationship, but this often comes with an intense time commitment and high financial cost. And if you're in some form of nontraditional relationship, finding a counselor with the right training and approach can be difficult. We wanted to create a relationship maintenance tool that would give the most bang for your buck, offering the most benefit for the least cost.

Road to Your First RADAR

Now let's get to the heart of the matter: the actual RADAR itself. This section is an overview of what you can expect from your very own RADAR session. These sessions will evolve over time. A couple's first RADAR may look extraordinarily different from their tenth or fiftieth RADAR. The important thing is to work together to build a safe space where each of you can be honest and direct while also being kind and nurturing. A RADAR will not always be easy or comfortable, but the goal is to work toward bringing a new level of intimacy and healthy communication to the relationship. We recommend choosing a nice setting for your first RADAR. Get cozy on the couch with plenty of blankets and pillows. Or go for a long walk together outside. If it feels right, you can even hole up at your favorite café. Honor this time that you are intentionally dedicating to your relationship; it truly is a special occasion!

RADAR:

Review
Agree the Agenda
Discuss
Action Points
Reconnect

R IS FOR REVIEW

The first part of the RADAR is to review the past month (or week, or however long it has been since your last RADAR). If this is your first regularly scheduled check-in, start by examining your previous month together. Once you are old pros at this, you'll know that the first step is to whip out your subsequent calendars or note-taking devices and recall important moments since your last RADAR took place. Did any family or friends come into town to visit this month? Was there an anniversary or important event? Did someone get a promotion or get laid off? Did a child get a particularly good grade at school or receive detention? Did the two of you have an argument? Get both the challenging and the jubilant times out on the table. Take notes on what you might want to recall for the steps ahead. The moment for discussion will come, but taking the time to look over what occurred since you last had a RADAR will help jog your memories and remind you of important moments during this time individually and as a couple.

A IS FOR AGREE THE AGENDA

We've come up with eleven important categories that most people will find crucial to discuss on a regular basis. Some of these topics may not pertain to everyone, and you may find that you want to add your own. Experiment with bringing up a particular topic for one RADAR and see if it's a relevant agenda point to add for subsequent RADARs. For your reference, we like to use the following topics and have included a few example questions for you to think about when you discuss each of them:

- **Quality Time**—How much time are we spending together? Do we want to spend more or less time together? If we live together, how often do we get out of the house or go on dates? How often are we sharing novel experiences together?

- **Sex**—Are we happy with the amount of sex we are having? Are there new and exciting things we would love to try? What are our feelings around sex with each other? Do we each have any baggage around sex? Are there triggers or specific ways that we need to make sure to be gentle with one another? If you or your partner are asexual, this could also be a question about the other ways you explore intimacy.

- **Physical & Mental Health**—Have there been any recent health issues? Were you ill in the last month? Are there chronic health concerns each of you should be updating the other on? What is the state of your mental health? Are either of you on new medications or exploring therapy? How are they working out?

- **Other Partners & Friends**—This is a good place for those in nonmonogamous relationships to get their partners up to speed on the other people they are spending time with. If this does not apply to you, discuss friendships or other important relationships in your life. How are your other relationships going?

Are there big life events that might affect your other relationships? Has a breakup happened? Have you been on dates with new people? How is your best friend doing? How often are you seeing them?

- **Fights & Arguments**—Did we have a particularly difficult argument that still needs to be resolved? If we successfully resolved a fight, is there anything we could learn from it? How are we approaching our communication around disagreements? Are there things that we could be doing differently or better? Are there patterns that we see in our arguments that we need to address?

- **Money**—Are there things that we are saving up for? Are there debts that each of us are working to pay off? How is that progress going? Is someone anticipating a large purchase or expense in the near future? Are we each approaching our attitudes about money in relation to each other in a healthy manner?

TACKLING CONVERSATIONS ABOUT MONEY

A lot of folks freeze up at the prospect of having a frank and forthright conversation about money with a partner. Whether you have been financially entwined for years or you're just starting to get to know about a new partner's financial situation, many people find this an awkward topic.

"To improve at discussing money, you need to work on empathy within yourself as well as your communication approaches," says Hadassah Damien, financial strategist and creator of Ride Free Fearless Money. Damien offers these tips for upping your game when talking about finances.

- Start small. "A practice of friendly, low-stakes conversations can ease money talks in general," says Damien. "Try discussing how to split a small food or entertainment cost. Approach it with genuine curiosity about how the other(s) might want to split it."

- Check yourself. "Generate equanimity: adjust if someone else's financial reality isn't as abundant as yours. Don't brag about tickets to Europe if the other partner's budget is a local road trip," suggests Damien.

- Don't take it personally. "If it's you who feels tender, practice not making it personal when someone else is talking about money," Damien recommends. "Find something you can learn from in their experience—it can reduce the sting of difference."

- **Work & Projects**—How is our work life going? Are we balancing our daily lives in conjunction with our work? Are there exciting opportunities or projects on the horizon? Is work a constant stressor? How is your relationship with your coworkers or bosses? What personal projects or hobbies are you working on?

- **Future Plans**—This can cover a wide range, including upcoming travel, anniversary plans, personal aspirations, or comparing visions of what the future of the relationship might hold. What would be a delightful way to make your next anniversary special? What do you and your partner dream about? What do you hope for next year? Are there any small-scale travel plans you want to make, like a day trip or hike? Any larger travel plans you want to start working on?

- **Family & Chosen Family**—May include kids, relatives, parents, extended relations, or chosen family. How are our kids doing? How are our parents doing? Do we need to discuss eldercare for any aging relatives? Do we have people coming to visit in the near future? Are there family members involved in holidays coming up? What kind of emotions come up when we discuss each other's family members or our own?

- **Household**—What does the distribution of labor look like if the two of us live together? Are we happy with the state of the household? Is one of us messy and the other quite neat? Are there renovations or household projects that we need or want to accomplish in the near future? If you don't cohabitate with your partner, this is a good opportunity to discuss how the two of you share your respective spaces. Would you feel more at home if your partner cleared out some drawer space for you in their closet? Would it be helpful if your partner occasionally picked up the grocery tab when you've been hosting and cooking?

- **Your Choice**—Always be sure to include any topics that are important to you and your relationship that are not covered in the list above.

D IS FOR DISCUSS

It's time to discuss each of the topics that you have laid out for the agenda. Even if a particular topic is not a problem area, still take some time to touch on it at least briefly. For each agenda item, it can be helpful to share at least one thing that you feel is going well in addition to one thing that you'd like to work on. If everything is fantastic for a particular topic, don't skip it! Take a little time to celebrate that together.

It's important to give yourself enough time during the discussion portion of the RADAR so that you can go in depth into the topics that need extra care. This might mean that you will need to take breaks during your discussion, especially if there was a topic that was particularly challenging or if something caused the two of you to get emotionally heated. This is a great place to incorporate all your best communication skills, especially all the tools covered earlier in this book! We also recommend checking out the sections on HALT, NVC, and I-messages in the Extra

Tools section. A lot of different emotions may arise during the discussion portion, and that's okay. In our experience, the same RADAR may bring up frustration, sorrow, awkwardness, excitement, arousal, and even raucous laughter.

A IS FOR ACTION POINTS

As you and your partner discuss, you may uncover new understanding, illuminate previously hidden areas of frustration, and dig into some much-needed problem-solving. A great way to solidify new knowledge or intentions is to create action points. Creating specific and achievable action points is vital in ensuring the two of you are moving forward and minimizes the risk of hitting a common relationship dead end: where both parties acknowledge a problem, but no one actually *does* anything about it.

When creating action points, it's important to incorporate language that is specific, realistic, and easily understood. Once time has passed, and you sit down for another RADAR, check in on your past action points during your review time to see how well you have achieved your goals. If you or your partner are struggling to execute on an action point, it may need to be tweaked or removed entirely. Not every discussion topic will need an action point. You might end your RADAR with no action points at all, but generally you'll want to have at least a couple tangible things to do during the next month, even if they are small and easily accomplished.

ACTION POINTS: CLEAR? SPECIFIC? ACHIEVABLE?	
INSTEAD OF THIS . . .	TRY THIS!
Phil will try to be more pleasant when Oscar's mother is around.	If Oscar's mother says something offensive to Phil, he will politely leave the room. Oscar will back him up if questioned.
Oscar will be better about initiating sex.	We'll pick out two evenings a week for sexy date nights and schedule it in the calendar. Oscar will commit to sending Phil some flirty text messages during the workday on those days.
We'll go on more fun dates.	We'll take turns scheduling and planning one really fancy night out a month. Phil will pick out the activity and dress code for this month's night out.
We'll be smarter about money this month.	Oscar will draw up a set budget for "fun" spending for us to try out. Once that money is spent, no more for the rest of the month. We'll reevaluate at our next RADAR and adjust the budget if needed.

R IS FOR RECONNECT

And finally, the fun part! It's time to reconnect to your partner! After a long and sometimes challenging RADAR, nothing is better than having a little special time to show your partner how much you care about them and how grateful you are that they went on this journey with you. Jaime Gama, psychotherapist and creator of Gotitas de Poliamor, stresses just how important this step is. "'We need to talk' can be a scary sentence. It is associated with fear, since even if we manage to get the conflict resolved, there can be an emotional hangover of 'What now?' The reconnecting phase of the RADAR allows partners to move back into a safe, loving place where the relationship is more than a conflict, a disagreement or 'a talk,'" says Gama. "As my clients navigate ethical nonmonogamy and find themselves overwhelmed with exploring this new dynamic, RADAR is a guide that allows them to know there is a wonderful rainbow of connection at the end of the storm."

After finishing up action points, a nice reconnect may involve verbally expressing appreciation to your partner for how they conducted themselves during the RADAR session. Praise each other for what went well. Even if there were disagreements, it's important to acknowledge your partner's feedback during those challenging moments. Be specific and thank them for taking the time to improve intimacy and work toward better communication skills.

After that, it might be fun to do an activity with your partner! Make a lovely meal, go out to discover a new type of cuisine together, play some video games, go for a walk, or even have some sexy time. The reconnection part of RADAR is the lovely cherry on top of the delicious sundae that is your monthly relationship check-in. Relish the feeling of a job well done!

Phil and Oscar's RADAR

After learning about RADAR from the *Multiamory* podcast (Episode 147), Phil asked Oscar if they could try it that weekend. At first Oscar was hesitant, and he worried that Phil just wanted to complain and tell him all the things he was doing wrong. However, after learning a little more about RADAR and getting assurances from Phil that he simply wanted them to have a less stressful way of talking about important things together, they agreed to give it a try.

Their first RADAR ended up taking almost four hours, which felt a bit overwhelming, but while processing, they started to realize how many little things they hadn't previously been able to discuss calmly and objectively. This included Phil's discomfort with Oscar's family, Oscar's feeling of neglect when Phil would overwork himself, the amount of time they spent together, their sex life, and their long-term dreams. Phil and Oscar discovered new things as well, including both of them craving quality time together off the couch and away from the TV, something neither had previously brought up. And Oscar learned from a slightly embarrassed Phil about some things he'd been curious to try in the bedroom.

When it came to Phil's work, they were able to discuss how it made Oscar feel when Phil was too focused on his deadlines to commit to quality time with him. It was a difficult conversation, but they made more progress on coming to a resolution than ever before. In the end, they decided to try having a quick conversation at the start of each week so that Oscar could know in advance how busy Phil would be. They still weren't sure if this was the final solution, but they decided to give it a try for the next month and then adjust after their next check-in if necessary.

The issue with Oscar's mom was trickier. They didn't get to a decision on their first RADAR, but they did finally have a chance to talk it through when they were both present and focused on the conversation. Oscar was able to express his mixed feelings about being close to his mother while also realizing that he had trouble speaking his mind around her or standing up for his relationship. Phil was able to explain his own baggage around a partner's parents slowly poisoning their relationship, and his fears that Oscar would eventually leave him. This first RADAR was a good starting point to better understand each other, but they realized this particular conversation would take a longer time to resolve. Luckily, they were both dedicated to continuing their RADARs and committed to supporting each other and working as a team to resolve issues together.

Lex and Rob's RADAR

Outside observers may think that having an intentional check-in must mean the relationship is high conflict or unhappy. In reality, RADAR creates an environment that helps to foster *actually* low-conflict relationships, not just conflict-avoidant relationships. As an example of this, let's go back to Lex and Rob.

Rob had been feeling uneasy about the gradual change he had seen in Lex during the years they had been together, so when he heard about RADAR on the *Multiamory* podcast, he suggested that they give it a try. This caused Lex to immediately go into fear mode. They were terrified that Rob was insinuating that he was going to break up with them, or that he had some really serious problems he wanted to discuss. It took a lot of assurance from Rob that he simply wanted an aid to strengthen their relationship.

Their first RADAR was fairly short and didn't change or address the underlying conflicts they had been avoiding. Lex's desire for harmony meant that they failed to bring up many of the things that were bothering them. It was difficult for them to even name anything they found wrong with the relationship. Lex had become so good at ignoring and deprioritizing any issue that they were hard to recall if they weren't confronted with them at the time.

A few more months passed where the couple continued to incorporate RADAR into their lives. Rob did his best to create a safe space where Lex could bring things to his attention without him reacting defensively. Over time, Lex started to test the waters and bring up small things, such as the sword hanging in their living room that made it feel less like a relaxing haven and more like a dungeony game room. As Rob continued to be receptive and gentle, Lex was finally able to bring up some of the bigger issues underneath the little ones, like their overwhelming fear of being selfish and how that led them to concede to him in discussions rather than express their own opinions. Rob also came to realize how his normal way of debating ideas could end up steamrolling Lex, even if that was never his intention.

For Rob and Lex, incorporating RADAR into their lives was not a quick fix but something that unlocked a much deeper understanding of each other's inner worlds and allowed them to discuss the differences they had. By committing to a regular check-in, they were able to slowly, gently but effectively transform their communication patterns.

Special Perks of the Nonmonogamous RADAR

Much of the work of *Multiamory* has been to "translate" mainstream relationship-health concepts and tools to be applicable and effective for a wide variety of nonmonogamous relationships. When Alanna Irving's blog post on applying agile scrum to relationships first caught our attention, our initial questions were related to nonmonogamy: Could this be helpful even in relationships that weren't on the escalator to marriage, kids, and beyond? Might this be a solution to the infamous communication overload that so many people experience in nonmonogamous relationships? Is it sustainable to maintain multiple check-in conversations with multiple partners? Our desire to get to the bottom of these questions was what motivated a long period of experimentation, tweaking, and getting feedback in order to create a tool that focuses first and foremost on nonmonogamy and nontraditional relationships, rather than including them as an afterthought. RADAR has been specifically developed to carry some specific perks for people in nonmonogamous relationships.

PERK #1: IT CREATES A SAFE CONTAINER FOR DISCLOSURE

Pop Quiz: You and your new partner, August, have reached a point of emotional intimacy in your relationship where you're ready to say, "I love you." What a milestone! You want to update your other partner, Camille, on the fact that this new relationship is escalating and have a discussion about what that may mean for the two of you (if anything). However, you also know that Camille has been having a rough week after going through a recent breakup. When is the right time to bring it up?

A. Right after Camille has finished crying on your shoulder about what a bad communicator her ex Steve was.

B. Once we've polished off the entire bottle of wine.

C. Text her at work as soon as the "I love you" happens.

D. Never. I'm terrified by the possibility of a reaction, even if I didn't do anything wrong.

The correct answer is E) NONE OF THE ABOVE, YOU SILLY BILLY.

This is a struggle that many nonmonogamous relationships face. "Issues about disclosure about other relationships are extremely challenging, since it is difficult for each individual to know what they really want to know about their partner's other partners," says therapist Kathy Labriola. "And even when someone knows exactly what disclosure they want, their partner(s) may not be willing to provide it, or may feel that their privacy or the privacy or their partners is being invaded. And you may feel very comfortable with a certain level of disclosure in one situation but feel a need for much more (or much less) information with another partner, because of the complex constellation of different feelings and fears engendered by particular partners and relationships."

In psychotherapy, the term *container* is often used to describe a dedicated space and time for doing some kind of emotional exploration, work, or processing. It is sometimes called a "frame" or just a "space," but the purpose is to create an environment that is different from daily life. In therapy, the container exists to differentiate the type of conversation and the type of emotional work you may do in the session, which has a clearly defined start and end point. Similarly, when we set aside dedicated time to have a RADAR check-in, rather than relying on spontaneous discussions, we are mentally making a container where we both agree to communicate honestly and vulnerably, while also making it safe for our partner to do the same. This container can allow us to speak with our partners much more deeply than we otherwise could during our normal lives with other emotions and concerns vying for our attention.

The main benefit of RADAR to nonmonogamous folks is that it offers a clear time and space for sharing with each other about what's going on in other relationships. This is important, because few of us have been given social scripts for that particular topic. In the absence of models to follow, many people fall to the extremes:

disclosing far too much information or far too little information, disclosing far too frequently or far too infrequently. Many people experience anxiety regarding when and how to share updates about other relationships, especially if this has already been a point of contention in the past. When there's a mutually agreed-upon space and time for giving state-of-the-union updates, much of the anxious guesswork is eliminated. "I've watched countless nonmonogamous clients feel immense relief in discovering the ways RADAR provides structure and guidance to emotionally activating conversations. Not only does the structure offer a framework for connective communication, it is uniquely reflective of the nonmonogamous experience in a way that makes my clients feel mirrored and represented," says Casey Tanner, sex therapist and creator of the @queersextherapy Instagram.

You and your partners will have to do the work of deciding what kind of updates are appropriate and necessary to share. We can't tell you exactly what that is, since it will be unique to your situation. As much as possible, we recommend prioritizing consent, respecting privacy, and infusing kindness and empathy into the conversation. There also may be certain updates and disclosures that you and your partners agree to share as soon as they come up, so don't feel restricted to only discussing updates during a RADAR. It's okay to talk about things as they come up. Labriola offers this advice: "Proceed slowly and with caution, and don't hesitate to modify your agreements as your needs evolve over time."

PERK #2: IT CAN BE A DRIVING FORCE BEHIND BUILDING RELATIONSHIPS WITH INTENTION

Choosing nontraditional relationships means choosing intentionality. There's no more relying on defaults and assumptions about how a relationship is supposed to work, and there's a whole new world of potential human connection. We find that RADARs and other relationship check-ins support the work of creating intentional, caring relationships that serve each person involved. A RADAR can be a great place to start when you and a new partner are figuring out just what kind of relationship you want to form together. Are we ever interested in combining finances or living together, or are we intending to keep that off the table? Will there be sex in our relationship? What amount of time is each of us willing or able to give right now? Asking these questions at the beginning of a relationship (and circling back to them when appropriate) is fundamental if you have multiple relationships at varying levels of entwinement, which leads us to the next perk:

PERK #3: NONNORMATIVE RELATIONSHIPS WELCOMED

Although the agenda topics can include talking points that are often associated with traditional, nested relationships (money, household, kids, etc.), RADAR was designed to be scalable to fit the scope of your relationships as they are. That means that even if you and your partner never intend to coparent together, or if you've chosen a romantic but nonsexual relationship, or if you're choosing a primarily kink-oriented connection with no intention of introducing one another to your families, you can still have a RADAR.

Customize your RADAR to fit the relationship that you are in today. That means that certain agenda items may be swapped out, or the length and frequency of your RADARs may be vastly different. For instance, you and your kinky comet partner (a person who may show up in your life briefly and then come around again after a period of time—like a celestial comet) may swap out the "household" topic for talking about Dom/sub dynamics, and instead of a monthly RADAR, you may choose to check in only once or twice a year.

Some listeners have even introduced RADARs as a regular check-in for their triad or quad. We recommend budgeting more time as you add more people, and be sure to customize the agenda to focus on what's relevant to the whole group.

BONUS PERK: RELATIONSHIP ANARCHISTS UNITE!

Relationship anarchy is the practice of applying anarchist principles and values to personal relationships. There are many different ways to practice relationship anarchy, but for many people this means disallowing external social pressures from defining their relationships, instead letting the people in the relationship decide for themselves how the relationship should function. Many relationship anarchists also choose to reject prescribed relationship hierarchies that dictate that any and all romantic partners must come first, taking care to prioritize friendships, family relationships, and other connections. We've found that RADARs work well in this context, too! There is nothing stopping the relationship anarchists out there from having a regular check-in with any important connection: your roommate, your coparent, your kids, and more. If this sounds totally wild to you, consider giving it a try. RADAR: it's not just for romantic relationships!

Troubleshooting

My partner is resistant to doing a regular check-in. How do I make the pitch for RADAR?

Before suggesting a RADAR to your partner, spend some time getting curious about your own desires and motivations. The homework assignment at the end of the first chapter of this book might be a good place to start. What are you longing for in your relationship? It could be a sense of closeness, a desire to feel safe and intimate while sharing vulnerable feelings, or a sense of ease that comes from knowing there's a time set aside to tend to the relationship. Establishing a regular check-in may just be one piece of something bigger that you're hoping for in your relationship. Knowing what you want out of your relationship gives you a jumping-off point for opening up this conversation with your partner.

Once you've done that work on your own, here are some suggestions:

- Highlight the positive things you're wanting rather than the negative things you're hoping to avoid or fix. "I'm hoping we can carve out time in our busy lives to take care of us" lands differently than, "I want us to stop getting so caught up in our own day-to-day shit that we neglect each other."

- Avoid criticism of your partner's behavior, feelings, or actions. "We need to have a check-in, because you are so conflict avoidant I can never bring anything up" is unlikely to be well received.

- Don't try to sell your partner on RADAR when

you're currently in the middle of conflict. Maximize your chances of being heard by waiting for a time when you're both relatively calm and feeling safe and connected.

- If your partner has concerns about establishing a check-in, listen, validate, and empathize without being dismissive.

- Collaborate together on lowering the hurdle. If your partner is unsure about a RADAR, is there a smaller, easier, simpler version of a check-in that they would be willing to try? At this stage, developing the habit of dedicated check-in time is more important than following the RADAR formula exactly. If you and your partner end up creating a monthly routine of spending just twenty minutes reflecting on what felt positive between the two of you that month and never end up doing a full RADAR, that's still a win!

This process takes too long! Is there any way to make it more time efficient?
While much of our Western culture prioritizes maximizing efficiency at every possible turn, your relationship health is not a good place to be cutting corners. However, a RADAR that regularly stretches to four, five, or upward of six hours is unlikely to be sustainable. Here are some guidelines for managing time:

- Budget at least two hours if you're having a RADAR on a monthly basis. A weekly, biweekly, or quarterly RADAR may need more or less time, accordingly.

- First-time RADARs tend to take longer, especially if there is a lot of unresolved relationship history. Plan ahead to honor your initial attempt at trying out this ritual with plenty of time and space.

- If you or your partner have a tendency to be long-winded, agree on an amount of time to dedicate to each agenda item. Set a timer for each topic or for each speaker. If your minutes run out, use it as an opportunity to practice pausing and evaluating together if this topic can be deferred to the next RADAR, or if you need to set up another day to continue the conversation.

- Before your next RADAR, jot down notes on the most important points or concerns for you. Bonus points for doing some exploratory writing to fully get your thoughts in order beforehand. (This is especially important for all you Spewers out there.)

- Experiment with time of day as well as location. You may find that you and your partner are more energized on weekend mornings, which allows you to get through your agenda faster than usual. You may also find that settling together at your favorite café allows you to focus better (and keeps both of you on better behavior) than at home.

- If you are genuinely short on time and cannot reschedule, agree on a briefer agenda by picking out the topics that are the highest priority to discuss. However, be honest with yourself about whether or not any particular topics are being consistently avoided.

As always, customization is your friend. You know best about your schedule, energy levels, and available time. That being said, intentionally dedicating a few hours to a check-in is better than unintentionally losing even more hours to unexpected blowups. You, your partner, and your relationship are worth the investment. "RADAR check-ins are most effective when practiced regularly, but with some bracketing around how long you will spend," says Tanner. "Whereas checking in 'as needed' can feel emotionally flooding and unpredictable, particularly for folks impacted by trauma, scheduled RADARs give members of a relationship the opportunity to plan for regulation, self-care, and relationship aftercare."

How do we maintain a consistent RADAR between juggling jobs, kids, and a billion other time commitments?
If you've already experimented with the suggestions above for managing time, but you're still having difficulties developing a consistent habit, here are some tactics to try:

- Find the interval between RADARs that works for you and your relationship. If it's difficult to set aside longer chunks of time on a monthly basis, experiment with dedicating one hour to a shorter check-in that happens on a biweekly basis. Or try out a quarterly RADAR.

- Connect your RADAR to another ritual or routine that already exists in your relationship. Dedeker and Jase have a set day each week for date night. Once a month, they dedicate one of those date nights to having a RADAR. No further decision-making or calendar juggling necessary.

- Attach a reward to your RADAR. Part of your reconnect step could be cracking into a new board game together. Or you could start your RADAR by getting takeout from your favorite, most indulgent restaurant. Or finally whipping out that new sex toy! Work together with your partner to uncover the juicy, exciting stuff that will be your pot of gold at the end of the processing rainbow.

Our RADAR just turned into a big fight!

We all have been there and done that. A RADAR that morphs into eight hours usually isn't the result of both people having such a splendid, enjoyable time processing together that they lost track of the time (though that could be possible). Running into intense conflict is the primary reason that a RADAR can stretch for several hours longer than planned. Here are some ideas:

- HALT (see the Extra Tools section) when emotions and pulses are starting to run high. It's a good practice to call a pause on yourself earlier than you think you need to. Going to separate spaces to take a breather and cool down may be all that's needed to come back to the topic with more kindness and focus. Or it may be a good time to table that partic-ular agenda item and come up with another dedi-cated time to revisit it.

- Add structure. If there are hot-button topics that are particularly difficult to get through, it may be a good opportunity to add some specific communication structure to your conversation. This may include reflecting, NVC, I-messages or one of the many other tools we discuss in the Extra Tools section.

- Experiment with switching up the order of the agenda. Is it better for you and your partner to get more difficult topics out of the way first while you have more energy before moving on to the easier stuff? Or is it better to knock out easy stuff in order to build momentum and connection before focusing on more difficult things?

- If you're running into conflict around the same topics over and over again, or if your conflict is frequently reaching explosive territory, consider getting some guidance from a counselor, therapist, or coach. A good professional will ideally arm you and your partner with tools, structure, and strategies that you can apply when you're on your own as well.

- Sometimes a fight is just gonna happen. Unfortunately, RADAR does not come with a conflict-free guarantee™ (neither do relationships). Opening up certain topics may also mean opening up old wounds, raw spots, and unexpected vulnerabilities that are uncomfortable to express yet necessary to explore. Each conflict is an opportunity to practice letting go of destructive communication in order to maximize understanding. Strive to bring your most productive, kind, and clear communication even in the midst of discomfort and challenging feelings.

I get anxious and/or my partner gets anxious before having a check-in.

Feeling wobbly before a RADAR is normal. In fact, all three of us have experienced at least some amount of anxiety before a RADAR, even after years of repetition. You may be carrying the dread of knowing that you'll be revisiting a bad fight you had earlier that week. Or you may just be feeling the anticipatory shakiness that comes from having to let your guard down and share your thoughts and feelings.

It doesn't help that many of us have been socialized to automatically assume that *intentional relationship talk* = *something bad is going on*. It's a common joke that receiving an unprompted text from your significant other that only says, "We need to talk" may be one of the more terrifying experiences known to humankind. Very few of us are used to seeing a check-in as something that could feel anything other than uncomfortable, much less positive and connective.

It's a big job to normalize intentional relationship communication on a grander social scale, but it starts with normalizing it within your own relationships. It is possible to incorporate gentle exposure to relationship check-ins by limiting the scale and focus of the talk as you are starting to develop the habit of having regular RADARs. If you are using RADAR correctly (having productive conversations, implementing effective action points, and feeling connected to your partner at the end), anxiety and dread may not completely disappear, but they should decrease over time. If negative feelings consistently dominate your emotional experience before, during, or after a RADAR, there may be some deeper problems within the relationship that need to be addressed.

Here are a few other strategies to try:

- Create the nest. Do whatever you can to help yourself and your partner feel soothed ahead of time. This could be a hot bath, meditation, gentle exercise, an orgasm, or more—any of these activities could be done joint or solo. You and your partner might take some time to build a literal nest for yourselves, bringing blankets, comfy clothes, and comforting scents. RADAR pillow forts are highly encouraged. One listener shared that they added a "preconnect" step at the beginning to help each other feel more loved and at ease.

- Make a ritual. Jumping into a RADAR right after you've been rushing to get home from a stressful day at work is unlikely to put you in a calm and collected headspace. Adding a ritual to mark the beginning of RADAR time can help to focus your mind and heart. This can be as informal as making a pot of tea together and talking over your intentions for this time. Or it could be as formal and woo-woo as you like, complete with crystals, candles, and an Olympic torch ceremony.

EMILY SAYS

My RADARs have moments of levity and laughter and some moments of anger and frustration. The truth is, I don't find RADARs to be easy, but I know how beneficial they are to my relationship in the long run. A little ritual that my partner and I have done for years is to bust out a glass of wine or a cocktail to sip on during the few hours that we spend tackling the many different agenda items. We don't do this to get drunk (that would be counterproductive to having an effective RADAR), but instead to have a nice little treat for the two of us to look forward to while we talk. I encourage you to go into your RADARs with a ritual such as this. That way you have something to look forward to while you are deep in discussion mode, in addition to maybe having an exciting activity planned for after the RADAR. Make your rituals specific to the two of you, and most importantly, try to have fun with them!

- If you normally deal with anxiety or an anxiety disorder, you know best what works for you and what's ineffective. The mental health section of the agenda is a great opportunity for you to share with your partner what you know about your anxiety and to collaborate on ways to reduce triggers leading up to a RADAR as much as possible.

- If you don't normally deal with anxiety, and you feel that you and your partner communicate reasonably well, yet the prospect of an upcoming RADAR

causes an unmanageable spike in distress, it's time
to get curious. It could be a trauma response linked
to something from the past or a prior relationship.
It's a good opportunity to explore and reflect with a
trusted friend or therapist.

**My partner and/or I are neurodivergent or have PTSD or other
mental health challenges. Having a RADAR sounds too daunting
or scary.**

While we have all experienced anxiety before sitting down for
our own RADARs, we recognize that anxiety may increase exponentially when paired with PTSD or other types of neurodiver-
gence. Talking about your relationship can be time-consuming
and arduous. In these instances, it may be easier to truncate
your RADARs and make them shorter, smaller, and thus more
easily digestible. It may also be best to have your RADARs
when you are your partner are generally feeling solid and steady
in your relationship. We wholeheartedly agree with what therapist Ruby Bouie Johnson says about how to approach significant
conversations with your partner: "Timing and presentation are
so important. When one has a loved one who has a depression, anxiety, trauma, or any other mental health concern, this
may change how information lands or is perceived. I encourage
'setting your partner up for success' with conversations. The
more you nurture safety, security, and stability in partnerships,
you are more likely to create positive and generative moments
in communication."

TIPS FOR CHALLENGING CONVERSATIONS

Additionally, Johnson provided us with an excellent list of best practices for partners who have trouble with challenging conversations. Even if you are neurotypical, these suggestions are fabulous reminders during emotional tumult or when facing difficult communication:

- Don't avoid conflict or hard conversations—it's okay to be uncomfortable and allow each other to practice managing self-soothing.

- Find strategies that work for you that allow you to self-regulate or co-regulate during conversations— and practice those when *not* in conflict. Practice will make it easier to access those tools when *in* conflict.

- Check your ableism—microaggressions, disenfranchisement, discrimination, unconscious biases, etc. These are the places where unwelcoming attitudes and antagonistic demeanors dwell. Explore how the infrastructure of relationships can be impacted by all the -isms.

- Don't pathologize your partner—PTSD or trauma are a part of a person's experience, but not all of a person. Pathology leads to enabling, belittling, and stigmatizing your person. This can lead to barriers for accountability and responsibility in partnerships.

- Compassionate curiosity—don't assume, jump to conclusions, or presume a person understands. Ask!!

- Be aware of your person's tender places (e.g., fear of abandonment, fear of rejection, not enough, need to be needed, etc.).

- Be aware of sounds, tone, body movement—sudden environmental changes can upend the best communication.

- Scheduling intentional time for communication is ideal.

CUSTOMIZE YOUR CHECK-IN

All three of us can attest to the power of the RADAR format, and we've seen so many of our listeners' relationships transform as the result of regular RADARs. But we will never make the claim that RADAR is hands down the best way to have a relationship check-in. The best type of relationship check-in is the one that works *for you and your relationship right now.* Whatever you whip up, we recommend including these key components for a successful check-in:

- It's easy to do on a regular basis.

- It's supported by an easy-to-remember and easy-to-follow formula or set order of events.

- It's flexible enough to adjust to the changing needs of human beings and busy lives.

- It can happen even when things are feeling great in the relationship.

Get cracking with your custom-made relationship check-in! And if you come up with a particularly juicy acronym for yours, please share the joy with us!

Takeaways

- A good relationship check-in happens regularly, can be customized, and creates a safe space for talking about difficult or uncomfortable topics.

- Customize your agenda so that you cover the topics that matter most in your relationship while also being sure that you're not avoiding or perpetually postponing topics that are awkward to talk about.

- Work together with your partner to create clear action points that will help keep you accountable and proactive.

- Reconnect with your partner after RADAR and acknowledge all the things they excelled at during the session.

- Communicate with your partner about the ways you can each make your RADAR an exciting ritual to look forward to every month.

For more information on RADAR, check out *Multiamory* Episode 147, "Relationship RADAR: Scrum 2.0" and Episode 315, "RADAR Troubleshooting."

RADAR Cheat Sheet

You can find a downloadable and printable version of this cheat sheet at Multiamory.com/RADAR

STEP #1: REVIEW

- Review what happened in your lives over the past month or so, or however long it's been since your last check-in. No discussion yet, just facts.

- Take notes if there are particular topics that arise that need to be added to the agenda.

- If you've had a RADAR before, discuss your past action points. Put incomplete action points on your agenda for discussion if need be. Celebrate the action points you successfully accomplished!

STEP #2: AGREE THE AGENDA

- Make a list of what you'll discuss.

- Decide on an order of agenda items that feels good for everyone.

- In addition to your custom topics, we recommend at least briefly touching on all of the topics listed below, even if there isn't anything *wrong*.

Quality Time	Money
Sex	Work & Projects
Physical & Mental Health	Future Plans
Other Partners and/or Friends	(Chosen) Family
Fights & Arguments	Household

STEP #3: DISCUSS

- Discuss each agenda item.

- A lot of different emotions may come up. That's okay!

- Use compassion, empathy, and active listening.

- If things get heated, it's okay to take a break to cool off.

- Be sure to include celebration of things that are going well, too!

STEP #4: ACTION POINTS

- As you discuss, collaborate on tangible, specific, and achievable action points to ensure you're both taking steps to grow and improve.

- Not every discussion topic will need an action point. You might end your RADAR with no action points at all, but usually it is helpful to have at least a couple.

- You can always check on progress and adjust or remove action points that are no longer serving you at your next RADAR.

STEP #5: RECONNECT

- Congratulate yourselves for completing a RADAR!

- Bring the discussion to a positive close with some reconnection.

- Find what feels safe and connective for you. This could include sharing appreciation for each other, giving compliments, jumping into a fun shared activity, exchanging loving touch, having sex, and more.

Use This for Good

We set out to write this book with the intention of helping people achieve better communication in their relationships. To us, good communication means the freedom to invest more time into the most wonderful aspects of a partnership—the intimate sideways looks that only the two of you share, the magic of experiencing something new and profound together, the fun of introducing a partner to a beloved family member, or the joy of feeling truly heard and respected. Our hope was that creating better communication would cut down on all the time spent dealing with misunderstandings, resentment, hurt, and anger. We hoped that these tools would help lay the groundwork for many relationships to develop, evolve, and grow. And then, just as we were finishing up the last touches on our book proposal to send out to prospective publishers, the pandemic shattered all normalcy. We didn't have a tool for that one.

We have collectively experienced a deep and painful trauma over the past few years. Our lives as we knew them have been fundamentally altered. Even if you were lucky enough to get through this time without losing a family member, friend, or significant other due to illness or simply a difference in beliefs, there is still an incalculable, incredible, profound sense of loss. In the midst of this devastation, the three of us wondered where our podcast and where this book would fit in. Was it frivolous to think that anyone would find solace or support in these resources? Would things like metacommunication, Microscripts, and RADAR truly matter in the time of COVID?

We were surprised to find the answer was yes. Despite the pain and despite the uncertainty, at the end of the day, we've found that our listeners, friends, and loved ones still ask many of the basic questions we've set out to answer through the tools in this book:

"How do I tell my partner I want to open up our relationship?"

"How can I fix the same fight I keep having with my roommate over who puts away the dishes?"

"Why does my girlfriend respond so poorly every time I try to give her advice?"

"How do I know if he and I are compatible?"

"I feel like I'm sinking. How can I get my partners to understand what I'm facing and what I need from them?"

If the pandemic has taught us anything, it's that what is most important and precious are the people closest to us. It's clear that connection and companionship is what makes life worth living, and it's what reminds us to have hope and optimism in the midst of pain and suffering. We hope you use what you've learned from these pages and channel it into creating the best connection and communication that you possibly can in your relationships and your communities. Use this for good. Use this for love. Use this for the people who you care about most. In the end, it's all that really matters. It's all we really have.

Extra Tools

Developing our own unique communication tools has been one of the most rewarding parts of creating and producing *Multi-amory*. There's truly nothing better than hearing that a tool has saved a listener's relationship, encouraged healthy communication for the first time, or established best practices to help a connection thrive. However, our tools and our podcast would not be possible without the work of countless others in the relationship communication and research field. The three of us are avid practitioners of many other communication practices established by doctors, therapists, authors, and researchers. This chapter is a collection of some of our favorite tools formulated by others as well as a few more tools of our own.

We routinely refer colleagues, listeners, and clients to these supplemental tools. We hope they will be helpful inclusions to your communication toolbox. If you are reading this chapter after completing the main portion of the book, you'll find expansions on some of the concepts we previously mentioned. Additionally, if a particular tool in this chapter speaks to you, we have included further resources to help you learn more. This is a great section to refer to if you need a quick refresher, or if you're craving some inspiration in the middle of a communication breakdown. We hope these tools will speak to you as much as they speak to us. Happy reading and enjoy!

THE TOOLS YOU WILL FIND IN THIS SECTION INCLUDE:

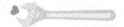

Apology Skills

Have you ever had someone apologize to you, but it just felt . . . insufficient? Have you ever given an apology that wasn't received as well as you had hoped? It's inevitable there will be moments of conflict, so learning how to give better apologies can go a long way in helping a relationship thrive, and aid in repair.

In *Multiamory* Episode 280, "Receiving and Giving Apologies," we spoke with Dr. Karina Schumann from the University of Pittsburgh, who studies apologies and conflict resolution. Schumann described the ingredients of a good apology as "an emotional mix of acknowledging what you've done, expressing remorse and regret for it, then giving signals that you're going to change it, that you're not going to commit that offense again." There is no magic formula for apologizing but these three factors, inspired by Dr. Schumann, are a good starting point:

- **Owning Your Actions:** Accept responsibility for what you have done. Avoid the urge to follow it up with justifications or excuses about why you behaved the way you did. While those reasons may be true and valid, they only serve to undermine the apology you are trying to give.

- **Expressing Regret:** Demonstrate that you feel contrition and wish that you had behaved differently. This is the difference between "I'm sorry you didn't like what I did" and "I'm sorry for what I did and that it hurt you." The first example shows no personal regret, while the second one is a much more effective apology template.

- **Offering Remedies:** It is not enough to apologize if the other person has no indication that you will work to make it right or behave differently in the future. The most important part of offering remedies is that you actually follow through on them. In some situations, there may be an easy remedy, such as replacing a lost or broken item, but more often things can't be replaced or fixed. In these cases, what matters most is finding a way to prevent this hurt in the future, which may involve some serious thinking on your part about how to ensure it won't happen again, or agreeing to an ongoing process of making amends.

The important takeaway is that there is more to an apology than just saying, "I'm sorry." In addition to knowing about the components of a good apology, it is also paramount that an apology is genuine and sincere. Expressing an apology without truly meaning it or failing to demonstrate a willingness to make future changes will amount to an insincere apology. Lastly, while this template will help you offer more effective apologies, they don't magically fix conflict, which is why it's so important to focus on communication, developing knowledge and awareness of others, and utilizing other techniques from this book to avoid hurtful situations whenever possible.

You can learn more about making good apologies on *Multiamory* Episode 280, "Receiving and Giving Apologies."

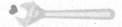

Attachment Theory and Attachment Styles

Attachment theory is a framework for understanding how people behave in relationships, especially long-term romantic relationships and parent-child relationships. The study of attachment theory has evolved over the past several decades. There are tons of resources about attachment styles, but here you'll find a basic breakdown of the concepts. Remember that your attachment style is not a sweeping proclamation of who you are as a person, nor is it a flawless prediction of how successful or unsuccessful your relationships will be. Use these concepts to help foster more understanding about what helps or hinders your feelings of safety in your closest relationships.

Attachment theory originally categorized people into three main styles of attachment, but many modern psychologists prefer to describe a person's attachment style using two scales: avoidance and anxiety.

AVOIDANCE

Attachment avoidance refers to how comfortable someone feels about getting close to another person, being intimate, or relying on another. Someone with high avoidance will be *less* comfortable letting themselves rely on a partner, or may feel uncomfortable with developing intimacy. On the other hand, someone with low avoidance will be *more* comfortable with those aspects of a relationship.

ANXIETY

Attachment anxiety is related to fears of being abandoned, neglected, or rejected by a partner. A person with low attachment anxiety is likely to be *less* fearful of those things happening, while people with high attachment anxiety tend to be *more* preoccupied with fears of rejection and being left.

When we view these two axes in a chart, we can then plot how high or low we are on the different spectrums and see which quadrant we fall into. There can be a lot of variation within a quadrant, but these labels may be helpful when looking for resources or seeking support. Below we will outline the different types of attachment within the avoidant and anxious scales:

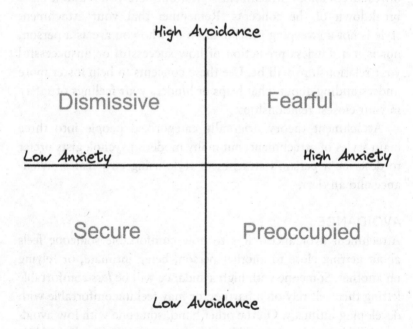

SECURE

Secure attachment is generally considered the ideal attachment style, combining a comfort with intimacy with a low fear of abandonment. It is important to note that while learning to craft a more secure attachment style is a worthy goal, having an insecure attachment style does not necessarily make a person less lovable or less able to have a rewarding relationship. Additionally, while a person may generally have a secure attachment style, they may exhibit behaviors of higher anxiety or higher avoidance more in certain relationships than in others.

PREOCCUPIED/ANXIOUS

A person with a preoccupied or anxious attachment style has higher levels of fear about being deserted or rejected by their partner but may be more comfortable with intimacy and reliance on a partner. Those who fall into this quadrant of the graph tend to be people pleasers, worry that they are not worthy of the relationship, and work hard to earn the love of the people in their lives.

DISMISSIVE/AVOIDANT

People who fall into the dismissive attachment quadrant, on the other hand, may have a hard time trusting others or letting anyone get too close. This fear of being vulnerable can be a significant challenge to developing loving, long-term relationships. However, people with dismissive or avoidant attachment may have an easier time making independent decisions and may not need as much support or reassurance from a partner as other attachment styles.

FEARFUL-AVOIDANT

This quadrant is high in both anxiety and avoidance, which often presents as a more deprecating view of both self and others. Not only do people with this attachment style fear that they are unworthy of love, but they have a harder time trusting that others will not reject or hurt them. As a result, people with a fearful attachment style will tend to avoid close intimate relationships while also craving relationships to help validate themselves, creating a difficult contradiction.

DISORGANIZED

This attachment style is characterized by inconsistent attachment patterns, often fluctuating between avoidant, aloof behavior and longing for intimacy and connection. This is caused by the contradicting desires for connection and self-protection. This attachment style is generally considered the most extreme of the insecure attachment styles and is often attributed to inconsistent caregivers or a history of abuse. Disorganized attachment can lead to a self-fulfilling prophecy of craving connection, perceiving threats that may not exist, and then withdrawing, leading to a relationship ending.

HEARTS

While a large part of our attachment styles is established during childhood based on our connection to our primary caregivers, it is possible to learn strategies for fostering more secure attachment in our relationships. In *Polysecure: Attachment, Trauma, and Consensual Nonmonogamy*, therapist Jessica Fern uses the acronym HEARTS to lay out strategies and skills that help to foster secure attachments:

> H—Here (being here and present with me)
> E—Expressed Delight
> A—Attunement
> R—Rituals and Routines
> T—Turning Toward after Conflict
> S—Secure Attachment with Self

If this is an area where you could use some help, we highly recommend checking out *Polysecure* to learn more about each of the skills, as well as exercises and suggestions of how to apply it in your life. You can also listen to our interview with Jessica Fern in *Multiamory* Episode 291, "Attachment Theory and Polyamory. "

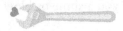

Bids

In its research on married couples, the Gottman Institute discovered a strong correlation between the happiness of a couple and how often they made and accepted offers of emotional connection with their partner. The term they coined for these offers is *bids*.

A bid is a verbal or nonverbal attempt at connection with a partner. When these offers of connection are accepted, the person who made the bid receives the message that their partner cares, appreciates them, and values the relationship. The Gottman Institute research shows that couples who are happy and stay together accept each other's bids around 86 percent of the time, while couples who subsequently broke up or were unhappy only accepted bids 33 percent of the time. Of all the factors they measured, this one was the most closely related to relationship success.

Making and receiving bids happens dozens of times a day. Learning to pay attention to our partner, recognizing bids as they are made, and responding by turning toward our partner is fundamental in creating a lasting connection. Because bids come in all shapes and sizes, they can take a little practice to recognize. Bids may even be surprisingly subtle, because making them big and clear carries a bigger risk of rejection. Here are a few examples of not-so-obvious bids:

- Your partner checks their text messages and lets out an audible sigh.

- In a tense moment, your partner makes a small joke to lighten the mood.

- While at a social event, your partner tries to catch your eye to give you a smile or blow you a kiss.

- While driving, your partner reaches over to put their hand on your leg.

- Your partner says, "I really want to watch that new Korean monster movie."

Researchers divided responses to bids into three categories:

- Turning Toward—Focusing your attention toward your partner and engaging with their bid.

- Turning Away—Either intentionally ignoring or unintentionally missing the bid entirely.

- Turning Against—Responding to the bid in a hostile or combative manner.

Each time we turn toward our partner, we are creating a positive emotional balance in our relationship. Each bid we miss subtracts from that balance, and turning against a bid is especially damaging. It happens in even the best relationships, but it is a surefire sign of destruction if it becomes a habit.

Even if we want to turn our partner down, it's best to do that in a way that engages with the bid, rather than ignoring or negatively rejecting. This can take some practice, but honesty and clear, kind communication is a great start. If your partner asks if you want to go for a walk while you're focused on a project, it is better to take a moment to acknowledge their offer and express that it is meaningful to you than to just say no or make an excuse.

To learn more about bids and the importance of turning toward your partner, check out *The Relationship Cure* by John Gottman. You can also listen to *Multiamory* Episode 168, "Communication Booster Pack."

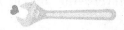

Consent and FRIES

The practice of consent has long been a predominant centerpiece of nonmonogamous, kink, and queer communities. With the prospect of many different emotional and sexual partners, it is vitally important to be able to clearly convey an enthusiastic yes or no to the advances of others. In our experience, having an awareness of consent can have a highly positive effect on all kinds of relationships, from traditional, long-term monogamy to workplace relationships and connections with friends. Consent isn't just about sex. You can have conversations about and give consent in more everyday and benign situations as well. Honoring consent shows that you have listened to your partner, that you respect them, and that you will work to ensure that they feel safe and loved. Planned Parenthood created the handy acronym FRIES as a way to remember five core principles of consent. While this model primarily focuses on sex, it can also be used outside the bedroom. The FRIES model states that consent is:

Freely Given—Consent should be given because you are excited about participating in a sexual act with another individual. Freely given means you are able to make clear decisions and are not under the influence of drugs or alcohol or being coerced or pressured into an act by another person.

Reversible—You can change your mind! Consent can be given, and then it can be taken away, even in the midst of a sexual encounter. If you are between the sheets, in the middle of taking off clothes, or even naked, if something doesn't feel right, you are free to reverse the consent you previously gave to your partner.

Informed—In order to give consent, you need to know all the details of your interaction and confirm your boundaries before getting sexual. This includes knowledge of things like STI status, deciding whether or not a condom will be used, and what types of sexual acts are okay or off-limits.

Enthusiastic—Can I get a HELL YES!? When giving consent, you should be excited and enthusiastic about the things you are about to do with a partner. Positive feedback, confirming you are okay with something before physically beginning an activity, and continuing an ongoing discussion about how each of you feels in the moment are all examples of enthusiastic consent.

Specific—Consent needs to be given for each specific act you are about to embark on. If you say yes to digital penetration, that doesn't necessarily mean you are also giving consent to oral or other kinds of sex. It should not be assumed that saying yes to one act automatically affirms another.

Even though consent discussions happen with more frequency in this day and age, it still can be a tricky concept to fully understand. For more information on another modality of consent, we recommend checking out Betty Martin's "The Wheel of Consent" and *Multiamory* Episode 272 with our friend Mia Schachter.

Demon Dance Battles, a.k.a. Pursuit and Withdrawal

In *Multiamory* Episode 275, "Demon Dance Battles," we covered pursuit-withdrawal patterns that show up in conflict. Dr. Sue Johnson, creator of Emotionally Focused Therapy (EFT), makes the case that while the content of a fight may change, the underlying emotional patterns often remain the same. She likens it to the steps of a ballroom dance—the music and the venue may change, but the choreography stays the same. Dr. Johnson calls these patterns "demon dialogues," but we couldn't resist roping in the choreography metaphor and decided to rename them demon dance battles. You're welcome, Sue.

These demon dance battles consist of two main behaviors:

Pursuing—moving attention and energy *toward* the other person. Pursuing could be as gentle as asking to talk things out with a partner, or it could be as destructive as leveling blame, blowing up, criticizing, steamrolling, or refusing to let the other person take a break or leave the conversation.

Withdrawing—moving attention and energy *away* from the other person. Withdrawing could look like choosing to take a break from a heated discussion, or it could be zoning out, defensiveness, stonewalling, minimizing the other person's feelings and concerns, or disappearing from the conversation for hours or even days.

Let's get the most important thing straight: *there is nothing inherently wrong with either of these behaviors.* We all experience alternating moments of seeking connection as well as seeking solitude. With a demon dance battle, however, these behaviors tangle into a toxic cycle. These are the most common patterns highlighted by Dr. Johnson:

The Find-the-Bad-Guy Boogie: Both partners show pursuing behaviors by being on the attack. Criticism and blame are hurled in both directions. There may be an endless back-and-forth in an attempt to prove beyond a doubt which side is right and which side is wrong.

The Protest Polka: One partner pursues, and the other partner withdraws. The "protest" part of this comes from the human tendency to protest against moments of emotional disconnection. The pursuer, desperately seeking safe connection, chases after the withdrawer, who shuts down in overwhelm or retreats in an attempt at self-preservation.

The Flight-and-Freeze Flashdance: Both partners turn away and withdraw. In this pattern, the relationship may seem peaceful and conflict-free on the surface. In reality, both partners may have emotionally disconnected long ago, or both may have internalized the assumption that conflict is unproductive, and therefore it's not worth it to engage in the conversation in the first place.

So what can be done about these demon dance battles? As psychiatrist Dan Siegel says, "If you can name it, you can tame it." Think about what sort of demon dance battle you and your partner fall into most frequently, and take the opportunity to metacommunicate about it together (ideally during a time when things are calm). Many EFT-trained therapists will have worksheets and other resources to help you map out all the steps of your particular fight choreography.

Once you have the clues that will help you recognize the pattern unfolding in real time, you have the ability to create a circuit breaker. Coming up with a way that either of you can name the pattern in the moment can help you to break out of it. Agree on what happens when the pattern gets called out. It could be a hug, taking three deep breaths, or taking a short break in separate rooms. Microscripts work great for this!

If you want to take a deeper dive, check out Dr. Sue Johnson's book *Hold Me Tight*, or listen to *Multiamory* Episode 228, "Pursuit and Withdrawal" or *Multiamory* Episode 275, "Demon Dance Battles."

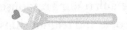

Fight, Flight, Freeze, Fawn

As a survivor of complex childhood PTSD, psychotherapist Pete Walker created a model for describing and understanding four basic defensive responses resulting from childhood abandonment, neglect, or abuse. The Four Fs, as Walker calls them, are a response of the brain's limbic system, which prompts an individual to ready themselves for survival. As you learn about these trauma responses, you may realize you don't exclusively adhere to only one. Most people default to a blend of two or more different responses depending on the situation. Each separate trauma response may manifest in a variety of ways, including the following:

Fight: Anger, control, and aggression may all be a part of the fight response. In a romantic relationship, if your partner says something that offends you, your response may include angry retorts, a desire to "win" a fight and not back down, acting aggressively, taking actions to control your partner and the situation, name-calling, contempt, or intimidation.

Flight: A flight survival response may present in many different ways. If your partner says something that upsets you, you might respond by leaving the room, avoiding eye contact, burying yourself in work so that you don't have to deal with the issue at hand, or engaging in substance abuse to flee from the problem. It also can result in being overly judgmental, a need for perfectionism in others and in yourself, and chronically busying yourself to avoid the magnitude of intimate relationships.

Freeze: Those whose default trauma response is freeze might subconsciously believe that people and relationships are dangerous and the safest option is to withdraw from intimate connections in general. It could also look like shutting down, zoning out, disassociating, or stonewalling. If this response is triggered while in a relationship, it might result in you resorting to total isolation or completely abandoning hope that a successful relationship is possible.

Fawn: People with this trauma response tend to engage in appeasing, people-pleasing, or self-abandoning behavior when faced with a triggering situation. You might be inclined to be overly agreeable toward your partner, work to minimize yourself so you don't "take up space," acquiesce to your partner's demands even if you're uncomfortable, or forfeit your own needs or boundaries.

Walker points out that those who had a fairly loving and positive experience with their parents and caregivers in early life will often have the capacity to healthily draw upon each of these responses in appropriate situations. Unfortunately, some of us did not grow up in safe and loving environments with solid support systems. If, after careful investigation of your upbringing and your response patterns in conflict situations, you find you have an unhealthy tendency to rely upon some of the behaviors listed above, it might be a good idea to find a trauma-specific therapist to uncover more insight.

For more information on fight, flight, freeze, and fawn, we recommend Pete Walker's book *Complex PTSD: From Surviving to Thriving*, as well as *Multiamory* Episode 316, "Fight, Flight, Freeze, or Fawn."

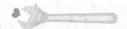

HALT (or HHALTDS)

The acronym HALT was initially used in recovery programs to help people manage their mental state in order to prevent relapsing during times of stress. Since then, it has also been used in many other areas, such as conflict management, decision-making, and communication. HALT stands for:

H—Hungry
A—Angry
L—Lonely
T—Tired

These are all mental and physiological states that make us particularly vulnerable to making poor decisions, including making unwise communication choices. Understanding HALT is key to minimizing out-of-control fights with a partner. A conversation, even one on a relatively benign topic, can be derailed if someone has an emotional reaction and responds in a hurtful way before they have a chance to think about what they are saying. This is much more likely to happen when one or more of the people involved are hungry, angry, lonely, or tired.

At *Multiamory,* we have added a few more vulnerable states to watch out for: horny, drinking, drugs, and sickness. This makes for the far less memorable and far more difficult-to-pronounce acronym HHALTDS, but we still think it's important to remember there are a variety of emotional and physiological states that can cause us not to behave at our best.

The great thing about HALT is that it serves as a reminder of what to do if you find yourself spiraling into conflict while in one of these states: stop. Check in to see if either of you might be hungry, angry, lonely, or tired (or horny, sick, or under the influence of substances), and then take a pause. Go eat, sober up, take a nap, masturbate, hang out with a friend, take time to feel better—whatever you might need to get into a better mental state to handle a potentially challenging discussion. While you are taking a break, it's important to use that time to restore yourself to a more balanced mental and physical state. This means avoiding things like venting to someone else, dwelling on your anger, complaining, being passive-aggressive, or otherwise keeping yourself overly emotional and unbalanced. Instead, take the time to take care of any physical needs, like eating or sleeping, and focus on something else for a while. Read a book, go for a walk, play a game, text a friend to let them know you care about them, meditate, work out, or do something else that centers you and rejuvenates your mind. After that, you'll be much better equipped to resume your previous conversation.

Calling a HALT in the middle of a discussion can feel like stonewalling or walking away, so it is important to explain that you need a break and to set a specific time when you can resume the conversation. This lets your partner know you do intend to continue, but you need to take care of yourself first. Depending on the situation, this could be anything from taking a twenty-minute walk to making plans to continue the following day. We have found that the pause should be a minimum of twenty minutes and ideally no more than a day, unless absolutely necessary, such as when recovering from an illness. Whatever you decide, be sure to communicate this in the most compassionate way possible, and then follow through on resuming the discussion. Often, you'll find that the next day it goes much better than it would have if you had tried to power through.

For more information on HALT, check out our multiple episodes on the subject, including *Multiamory* Episode 218, "I've HALTed. Now What?"

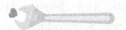

I-Message

When a discussion starts getting heavy, it's easy to get defensive and place blame on your partner. A good way to avoid this is to use an I-message to describe your feelings and desires while reducing feelings of shame or blame in the other person. The concept of the I-message was developed in the 1960s by Dr. Thomas Gordon in his work in play therapy. I-messages stand in contrast to the concept of a you-message, which usually begins with "you" and describes the feelings and motivations of the other person, often putting them on the defensive.

In most circumstances, saying something like, "I'm angry with you," may leave your partner confused as to what they did wrong, why you're angry, and what they can do to fix the situation. Simply stating a feeling isn't necessarily enough information to help your partner understand the reasons for your reactions. That's why Gordon created the "confrontive I-message" which is made up of three components in order to clearly convey a grievance to your partner. Those three components can be stated in any order and include:

1. A short description of the thing or behavior that you found to be inappropriate. In this description, it is important not to blame or accuse your partner.

2. The specific feelings you felt because of what happened.

3. The impact the behavior had on you.

Using I-messages can help you be more diplomatic in your approach while tactfully and clearly relaying an issue to your partner. Hopefully, this can introduce a component of problem-solving instead of creating a reason for your partner to get defensive. Rather than getting emotional and blaming your partner for something that they did, you might say:

- "I feel incredibly anxious when you stay out until 2 a.m. and don't call or text. I get worried about your safety and wonder where you are."

- "I felt jealous when you took your new partner to

that cool restaurant before we got to experience it. It reminded me we haven't been out on a fancy date in a while."

- "I feel really sad when we don't get enough family time. I want to make sure our daughter gets quality time with all of us together, and when we're too tired to play with her, I worry about her feeling sad, too."

We recommend practicing I-messages in a benign environment with your partner so you'll be old pros at it when a heated argument does occur. For more information on I-messages, check out the work of Dr. Thomas Gordon at gordontraining.com.

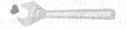

It's Okay to Break Up

This section doesn't have a convenient tool or snappy acronym. We just want to offer some simple reassurance in the form of a classic *Multiamory* adage: *it's okay to break up*. Yes, it's scary, inconvenient, disruptive, heartbreaking, painful, and potentially devastating. We have all been there. This especially goes out to those of you practicing some form of nonnormative relationship. It's easy to feel like the dating pool is too small, like your needs and desires are too weird, or that everyone around you will see you and your relationship style, gender identity, or sexuality as a failed choice because a particular connection didn't work out. On top of that, there are strong social norms that encourage staying in a decidedly bad relationship for the sake of longevity and commitment. All of us feel this pressure, and it can make the choice to end a relationship excruciating. We see you, and we share your pain.

Regardless of your relationship configuration, breaking up is hard to do. If you've been together for years, put in a huge amount of emotional effort, and entangled yourself financially, leaving a relationship may feel overwhelmingly disruptive and frankly more trouble than it's worth. This is known as the sunk-cost fallacy, and it's one of the many reasons why people tend to stay together even when the relationship is no longer healthy or happy. Additionally, you may recognize there isn't anything drastically wrong with your relationship, which therefore makes the decision to leave that much more difficult. After all, if your partner isn't outwardly abusive, you enjoy each other's company, and your parents love them, shouldn't you just try to work it out?

In some instances, however, you may be questioning what kind of behavior constitutes abuse. Claire Louise Travers, creator of Poly Pages, highlights the difference between abusive relationships and those that are simply not working: "As opposed to unhealthy or incompatible relationships, abuse is a persistent pattern of behavior, which takes away our power and control. Abuse tactics are more than physical or sexual violence, and include emotional manipulation, financial abuse, isolation, weaponizing privilege, and minimizing or denying abuse. Knowing these tactics can help us identify behaviors in our relationships and community. Abuse has the design, intent, or consequence of making you unable to leave a situation. So ask yourself, 'Can I step away from this?' Leaving an unhealthy or incompatible dynamic feels hard, but dread, fear, or isolation may indicate abuse is/has been present."

Here's the thing—a relationship doesn't have to be abusive for it not to be right for you. Even if you know your relationship

doesn't carry signs of abuse, a pile of negative day-to-day interactions may be a signal that moving on is the best decision for
both of you. Research from a longitudinal study conducted by the
Gottman Institute shows that you should ideally have five positive interactions with your partner for every one negative interaction. This is a fantastic metric to apply if you are questioning
whether or not your relationship is still serving you. Ask yourself, is the majority of the time I spend with my partner happy,
easy, and something I look forward to? Or do I find myself internally dreading our interactions, feeling as though I'm walking on
eggshells, or looking more forward to time away from my partner
than time with them?

An ending does not necessarily signal failure. Breaking up can
be the healthiest, kindest, and most mature way to transition into
the next phase of a relationship. A breakup can also create new
beginnings. Jase and Emily have found that their relationship is
happier, more stable, and closer than ever now that they are no
longer romantically involved. The years of care and commitment
they showed one another as romantic partners have transferred
over to help craft a wonderfully meaningful and secure friendship.
Even if you choose not to stay friends with an ex, a breakup can
allow you the opportunity to give thanks for all that your partner
and your shared experiences have taught you.

Because breakups can be so challenging, we recommend doing
everything you can to care for yourself, keep yourself safe, and
to get outside perspective in the form of a trusted friend, mentor,
or therapist. We also highly recommend *The Polyamory Breakup
Book* by Kathy Labriola or listening to *Multiamory* Episode 289,
"De-Coupling."

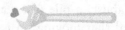

MOVIES

For the first few dates, it's easy for two people to gloss over some of the more nitty-gritty elements of what their specific practice of nonmonogamy looks like. Unfortunately, we've heard many stories of heartbreak and incompatibility when people find out after the fact they are not on the same page. Several years ago, there was a long list of "glass-ceiling questions" that bounced around the nonmonogamous community. These questions were established for people to really get to know the ins and outs of a potential partner's beliefs about relationships, and specifically how they chose to practice nonmonogamy. Essentially, these questions were meant as a filtration tool to expedite the process of finding someone whose style of nonmonogamy fit with yours. Because this list of questions had about sixty-four thousand different items on it, we gave it the *Multiamory* treatment and came up with our own handy acronym for getting to know the specifics of the other person's relationship style. If you want to learn more about a new partner, all you have to do is take them to the MOVIES! These are the important topics to hit early on in a new dating relationship:

MOVIES

Metamours
Openness
Veto
Intimacy
Events
Scheduling

Metamours

Who are my potential metamours? What type of polyamory do you and your partners tend to practice (i.e., don't ask/don't tell, kitchen-table polyamory)? Is there an expectation that metamours will be in contact with one another? Is there an expectation that we will need to have any sort of relationship with one another (friendship, acquaintance, or otherwise)?

Openness

How open and out are you to the world about your nonmonogamy? How comfortable are you with public displays of affection, appearing together on social media, or otherwise? Do your family or children know you are polyamorous? Your friends? Coworkers? If not, how does that affect your life and how you conduct your relationships?

Veto

Do you have a primary partner or practice hierarchy in your nonmonogamous relationships? Do you have rules in that relationship? Does your primary partner have veto power over other partners? Are there any other potential restrictions on your relationship, like a curfew, a limitation on which genders one or both of you are allowed to date, or any quota on number of partners or amount of time spent together?

Intimacy

Are you sexually active, and is sex a part of the relationships you want to have with potential partners? What are the safer sex practices that you incorporate into your nonmonogamy? Do you regularly get tested for STIs? Do you have boundaries regarding sex? What are some of your favorite ways, besides sex, to express intimacy to your partners?

Events

What kind of events are okay to attend together and what are off-limits? Are vacations something that you only take with certain partners? How about work functions, holidays with family, birthdays, play parties, or overnight trips?

Scheduling

How do you prefer to schedule upcoming dates? How much time do you have to dedicate to a new relationship? Do you use things like Google Calendar, and do multiple partners have access to this calendar? How much time might we expect to see each other during a typical week? Are sleepovers okay?

These categories are customizable and may or may not pertain to every type of nonmonogamous relationship. However, for many people, these questions will provide a great jumping-off point and a way to get you and your partner to think more critically about how you like to conduct your relationships. Dating and relationship coach Marie Thouin, PhD, offers additional question ideas to discuss with potential nonmonogamous partners. "First, I'd want to learn about what sparked their interest in consensual nonmonogamy, and what CNM means for them. Then, I'd be curious about how they've put their relationship philosophy into action: What obstacles have they encountered? How have they dealt with them? What have been their greatest learnings along the way? I'd also ask about what particular style(s) of nonmonogamy they are involved in, what preexisting relationship agreements they might have with existing partners, and how they generally prefer to communicate with lovers and partners. Finally, I'd discuss their emotional availability, their sexual desires and boundaries, and what support system (friends, mentors/coaches, community) they lean into when encountering relationship challenges."

For a more in-depth discussion on MOVIES, check out *Multiamory* Episode 133, "Six Questions You Must Ask Your New Partner."

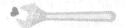

Nonviolent Communication and Clean Talk

Nonviolent Communication (NVC)—First coined and created by Marshall Rosenberg, NVC is a conversation structure that can be especially useful when discussing challenging topics. Ideally, NVC is done with one partner speaking for as long as they want without interruption, and afterward, the other partner will have an opportunity to do the same. These are the four main steps of NVC:

- State an *observation* of what happened, free of interpretation, accusation, or your own spin on what occurred.

- Express your *feelings* without applying your own story about what was done to you by the other person involved.

- State what you *need* from your partner or what your general needs are.

- Make a *request* that is not a demand or an ultimatum. Your partner should feel free to say yes, no, or to negotiate the request.

Example of a Clean Talk script:

"Yesterday you canceled our plans to go out to dinner two hours before we were supposed to get together. I felt hurt, because I had been looking forward to seeing you for weeks. I need to know that you value my time and this relationship. In the future, I would like you to let me know at least a day in advance if you need to cancel or change plans."

Clean Talk—Cliff Barry, founder of Shadow Work Seminars, originated Clean Talk, a means of healthy communication similar to NVC. These are the four steps that demonstrate Clean Talk:

- Relay simple, easy-to-understand *data* about an event or situation. This creates an opportunity to reexamine what happened during a disagreement.

- State your *feelings* about the event or situation without adding on additional stories about why those feelings occurred.

- Add your specific *judgment* about what happened in the situation. This is a good time to relay your story and thoughts to your partner and see if their interpretation is in line with yours.

- Relay what you *want* from your partner, or how you would prefer the situation to go next time.

Example of a Clean Talk script:

"Yesterday you canceled our plans to go out to dinner two hours before we were supposed to get together. I felt very hurt, because I had been looking forward to seeing you for

weeks. It made me feel as though you don't value my time or this relationship as much as I do. In the future, I would like you to let me know at least a day in advance if you need to cancel or change plans."

Similarities and differences between NVC and Clean Talk:
Both models use some form of *observation* to state what happened during an experience without drawing any specific conclusions about the other person's actions or rationale. Both models also require a statement of *feelings* without putting a judgment value on them or on your partner. Finally, both models provide the opportunity to make a *request* of a partner at the end of the session.

A key difference in the Clean Talk model is that each person is encouraged to relay *judgments* about the situation that occurred. The idea behind the inclusion of judgments is to add a level of understanding to the situation, as well as allowing your partner the chance to correct your judgment if it was inaccurate. Ideally these judgments are conveyed in a way that is not harmful toward your partner but instead offers some clarity as to why you are feeling a certain way.

NVC maintains that the person speaking can continue uninterrupted for as long as they want. Alternatively, Clean Talk is done in rounds and offers each listener a chance to respond once each section of the conversation is finished. This might be a beneficial tactic to use if a partner tends to get defensive or feel piled on when a criticism is leveled at them.

For more information on NVC, we recommend checking out *Nonviolent Communication: A Language of Life* by Marshall B. Rosenberg. If you want to learn more about Clean Talk, check out *Practically Shameless* by Alyce Barry or various Clean Talk Shadow Work Seminars online. We also cover this in depth in *Multiamory* Episode 241, "Five Ways to Suck Less at Communication: The Revival."

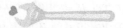

Putting Feelings into Words

So many of the tools in this book are for the purpose of enhancing your communication, making it easier for you to describe your needs, make requests, set boundaries, and express your feelings. But what about when your feelings are confusing, elusive, mixed-up, or if you've always struggled with putting your emotions into words? We've got you covered with two different techniques for attaching words to your feelings:

WHEEL AND DEAL

Researchers have spent a lot of time, money, and effort trying to determine the exact number of universal human emotions, producing results that suggest as few as five to as many as twenty-seven distinct emotions! In addition, many people have tried to map human emotion into an understandable formula. Enter emotion wheels.

If you google "emotion wheel," you'll find many variations on a similar theme—an extensive list of emotions, usually arranged into a circular shape. There is the Geneva wheel, the Junto wheel, and many others, but the one that most people are familiar with is the Plutchik wheel, developed by psychologist Robert Plutchik in 1980.

Having an emotion wheel on hand can not only help give you a list of feeling words but can help you map out different variations of emotional intensity, understanding the core emotion underneath, as well as determining all the different pieces of mixed or chaotic emotions. You can use an emotion wheel to see if any particular emotion label seems to fit what you're currently experiencing, then verbalize that to your partner. Or you might take some time asking questions to get more clues:

What might have been the catalyst for this feeling?
What are each of these feelings trying to say?
Is this feeling old and familiar, or does it feel new and novel?

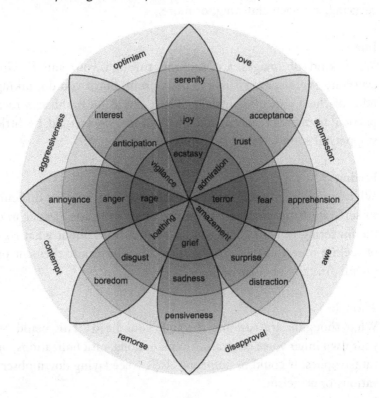

SIFT THROUGH IT

This is one of Dedeker's favorites! This tool was developed by psychiatrist Dan Siegel in his book *Brainstorm: The Power and Purpose of the Teenage Brain*. If it's good enough for teenage emotions, it's good enough for us. It all starts with the acronym SIFT—sensation, image, feeling, thought.

Sensation
What sensations are occurring in the body at this moment? This may include throat tightening, heart beating, muscles tensing or relaxing, stomach churning, or more.

Image
What kind of images are running through your mind? Not everyone experiences visuals in their brain, but if you do, taking note of them can offer insight. These could be flashbacks to a particular memory or an imagined future, or it could be little snippets of sound, touch, or familiar faces.

Feeling
What emotional sensations are inside you? This may be difficult to separate from physical sensation, but if you dive deeper into the fluttering in your chest, you can get curious about what sort of feeling tone the sensation carries. Is it fluttery excitement or dread? Anxiety or surprise?

Thought
What thoughts are running through your head? This could be your own inner voice generating explanations, rationalizations, or catastrophes. It could be someone else's voice laying down observations or criticism.

SIFTing works in many different scenarios, whether you are journaling, talking to a partner, or just having a moment of self-examination. Each element of SIFT may also feel interconnected in some way. Tracking those connections and how each element influences another can also offer valuable information about your own inner world.

You can learn more about these techniques, as well as more

on nonverbal techniques, in *Multiamory* Episode 348, "Transforming Feelings Into Words."

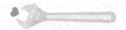

Reflecting

Reflecting is a simple yet surprisingly effective technique for increasing mutual understanding, particularly when the conversation is about something important. At its core, reflecting is a process of listening attentively and then repeating back what the other person said in order to ensure you understood it correctly. There are two main variations on reflecting that can both be useful at times: mirroring and paraphrasing.

Mirroring involves repeating back what the other person said using the same words (or as close as you can remember). This works best with shorter pieces of information or by mirroring just one key part of what they just said. When used well, this shows that you listened and paid attention to what was said, and it offers the other person a chance to clarify or elaborate on what they meant by it. If misused, however, it can come across as irritating or even mocking, so it is best used with intention. While it may seem like parroting someone's words back to them would be annoying, if you give it a try, you may find that people take to it surprisingly well, and that it can help encourage them to share with you. While mirroring can be effective at showing the other person you are actively listening, it is less effective at ensuring that you truly understand what they mean by those words, which is where the second technique comes in.

Paraphrasing is arguably the more advanced and more effective technique when it comes to establishing mutual understanding in a conversation. Paraphrasing involves repeating what you believe the other person is saying but using your *own* words. The power here comes from showing that you are not just listening but actively trying to understand the meaning. When paraphrasing goes well, it not only shows that you are paying attention but also gives the other person an opportunity to clarify their thoughts or make corrections if you came away with a slightly different understanding. As humans, we can't avoid processing information with a large degree of bias based on our own experiences and beliefs. Have you ever had a conversation where both of you felt you shared information and understood one another, but then weeks later you realized you both seem to have totally different memories of the conversation? This is an example of these biases at work, which reflecting and paraphrasing can help to minimize.

Paraphrasing is not without its challenges. If paraphrasing comes across as judgmental, accusatory, or minimizing, it can put the other person on the defensive and derail communication. For it to be effective, there needs to be a base level of trust and goodwill between you and the other person. For more information, check out the reflecting informational page at https://counseling.education/counseling/skills/reflecting.html.

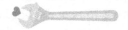

Repair Attempts

Conflict is a normal part of relationships, but conflict that spirals out of hand can soon rob a relationship of joy. Each person may have different triggers and hang-ups that can escalate conflict, but here are a few common signals that a disagreement may be starting a downward spiral:

- Difficulty focusing on one topic, bringing up past conflicts or hurts, switching subjects

- Interrupting each other

- Emotional escalation, such as feeling suddenly overcome by anger, sadness, anxiety, etc.

- Physical activation, such as heart rate increasing, breath getting faster and shallower, palms sweating

- Cyclical pursuit and withdrawal behaviors

- Expressing increasingly negative sentiments about yourself, your partner, or the relationship

Preventing this downward spiral of negativity is key not only to healthy conflict but to a healthy relationship. This is where repair attempts come in. A repair attempt is any statement or action that prevents negativity from escalating out of control, helps get the conversation back on track, and starts reestablishing the connection between you and your partner.

Much of the research on conflict resolution in relationships supports this. A 1995 study on marital satisfaction published in *Journal of Marriage and Family* found that relationship satisfaction is positively related to the frequency with which both partners resolve conflict constructively, using strategies such as agreement, compromise, and humor. On the flip side, relationship satisfaction was negatively related to the frequency of destructive conflict strategies, such as withdrawal or defensiveness.

In addition, Gottman Institute researchers found the happiest couples repaired at a much lower threshold of negativity than unhappy couples did. They also found what happens in the first three minutes of conflict sets the tone for the rest of the conversation. Three minutes!

So what do repair attempts look like in real life? Here are some examples, grouped into categories. We recommend having this list handy for the next time you find yourself in spiraling conflict. It may feel phony at first, but over time, you'll learn to hone your repair attempt skills and make them your own:

- **Disclosing feelings**
  "I'm feeling sad."
  "I feel sensitive about that topic."
  "I feel criticized. Can you rephrase that?"

- **Getting meta**
  "It seems like we've been misunderstanding each other's intentions for a while."
  "I think we're getting off track. Let's get back to talking about the real issue."
  "It sounds like it's difficult for you to fully listen to me when I'm upset, and I get upset when it seems like you're not fully listening."

- **Slowing down**
  "Let's slow down. I want to make sure I'm understanding."
  "I got a little carried away. Let me take that back and say it in a better way."
  "This is a difficult topic for me. Please give me a little patience."

- **Asking to stop**
  "I need to pause this conversation. Give me twenty minutes to cool off."

"I'm feeling overwhelmed and paralyzed."
"Can we stop talking about this for now? I need some time to think."

- **Finding agreement**
  "That's a good point."
  "I agree with a part of what you're saying."
  "Let's both make an effort to check in with each other about this."

- **Kind, playful humor**
  We can't tell you which silly jokes are going to land with your partner. The important part is to ensure that the humor is kind and reciprocal with no contempt or malicious intent. Whenever Jase says, "You really lost your cool," it makes Dedeker giggle, because inside jokes. But it works!

For more on repair attempts, you can check out *The Seven Principles for Making Marriage Work* by John Gottman. You can also listen to *Multiamory* Episode 288, "Repair Attempts."

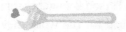

Switchtracking

Switchtracking is a term coined by Harvard Law School lecturers Sheila Heen and Douglas Stone in their book *Thanks for the Feedback: The Science and Art of Receiving Feedback Well.* *Switchtracking* is a term for one person changing the subject or switching to a different topic after receiving feedback from another person. This is what it looks like:

Person A: Why haven't you taken out the trash yet? I asked you an hour ago. I don't want to have to keep pestering you.

Person B: You always point out the things I *don't* do instead of appreciating all the work I *do* do.

Person A: But the trash is overflowing and starting to smell. Please take care of it.

Person B: I really hate how little you notice all the work I do around the house.

The argument continues, with each partner literally talking about two different subjects in the same conversation.

Switchtracking isn't necessarily a negative thing. Often two people will seamlessly change topics in a conversation or move onto a more important discussion point without conflict. However, issues can arise when the person doing the switchtracking is trying to stop a point of conversation from happening, or if each person chooses to dig in their heels and continue having two separate conversations at the same time. In the example above, Person A is trying to tell their partner to take out the trash and that they don't want to continue pestering them about it. Person B switches topics and starts to discuss how they feel undervalued for the work they do around the house. Both conversations may be valid and fair to have, but most likely, both can't effectively be discussed and resolved at the same time.

Switchtracking is incredibly common, and having an awareness of the pitfalls that can come from changing topics in a heated conversation is one of the ways you and your partner can learn to get back on track. Try to gently point it out the next time switchtracking happens in a conversation (Pro tip: It's easier if you're calling out your own switchtracking, rather than criticizing your partner). Give the two different conversation topics names, agree to stick to one in the moment, and set a time to discuss the other topic in the near future.

For more information on switchtracking, check out *Hidden Brain* Episode 1, "Switchtracking," *Multiamory* Episode 168, "Communication Hacks Booster Pack," as well as the book, *Thanks for the Feedback: The Science and Art of Receiving Feedback Well* by Sheila Heen and Douglas Stone.

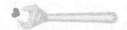

Values

Understanding your values is a fundamental part of creating good relationships as well as creating a good life. Human relationships and the twists and turns of life consistently expose us to new, unknown, and confusing situations. Our values are what help to guide us during these moments where there is no clear answer in the fog. These are just a few of the puzzling questions many of us have to tackle at some point in life:

- Should I stay in this relationship?

- Is it better to try something new or to stick with the tried and true?

- Is this an area where I can compromise, or should I stick to my guns?

- Can I forgive my partner for how they've hurt me?

- How do I communicate in a gentle, loving way even when my blood is boiling?

But what even are our values? We like this definition from a 2017 meta-analysis of multiple studies on values, published in the research journal *Nature Human Behaviour*:

"Personal values are defined as broad, trans-situational, desirable goals that serve as guiding principles in people's lives . . . Values refer to what is good and worthy."

Our values are influenced and shaped by many different forces, including your broader social group, the microculture of the family you grew up in, the principles of the religious organization that you're a part of, as well as direct influence from your caregivers and peers. That being said, values can shift and change over time, and sometimes it's not immediately apparent what your values are today.

There are about a kajillion different exercises out there for determining your values. We condensed and modified our favorite exercise, originally from MindTools.com:

Identify some times in your life that you were the happiest. What were you doing? Were you with other people? Who? What factors were contributing to your happiness?

- Identify some times in your life when you felt proud. Why were you proud? Did other people share your pride?

- Identify the times when you were the most fulfilled and satisfied. What need or desire was fulfilled? How and why did this contribute meaning to your life?

- Looking over the things you wrote, are there any common themes? What has been most important to you? This is the stage when it can be helpful to consult a list of value words—(for example, empathy, independence, freedom, consistency, love, joy) and pick out as many or as few that make sense, then condense into a list or hierarchy from there.

- Reaffirming—when I look at this list of values, do they make me feel good about myself? Am I proud of my top three values? Would I be comfortable and proud to tell these values to people that I respect and admire? Do these values represent things I would support, even if my choices aren't popular and they put me in the minority?

For more about values, check out *Multiamory* Episode 319, "What Are My Values?"

Acknowledgments

It takes a village to raise a podcast baby, and an even greater one to bring a podcast book into the world. We deeply appreciate the community of people that has sprung up around *Multiamory*. This work would be impossible without you. In particular, we would like to thank:

Our audio editor, Mauricio Balvanera. We are eternally grateful for your hard work and eternally apologetic for all of our mistakes that you have to clean up.

Our production assistants, Carson Collins and Rachel Schenewerk. We majorly lucked out in finding both of you. You both bring a particular blend of dedication and good humor that inspires us to keep going.

Our research assistants, Em Mais and Dr. Keyanah Nurse. Thank you for your sharp analyses, insightful opinions, and speed-reading skills. Having you on the crew has elevated both the podcast and this book.

Our agents, Michael Bourret and Uwe Stender. Thank you for sharing our eagerness for making this book a reality, and thank you for supporting us on every step of this process.

Our publisher, Cleis Press, and especially our editor, Rene Sears, for choosing to bring this book into the world and helping us refine and clarify our ideas so that everyone can benefit from them.

Our network manager, Cameron Poter, and the whole Pleasure Podcasts team. Thank you for your inspiring team spirit, advocacy, and solidarity.

Our social media management and brand consultant team, Britney Walters, Pierre Walters, and Bethany McKinzie. Thank you for keeping us lookin' good.

Thank you to our sensitivity reader, and thank you to our early readers, Phoebe Philips, Brandi Vos, Keri Rico, and James Rappaport. Your honest thoughts, critique, and encouragement made this book better.

It is impossible to list everyone who has contributed to *Multiamory* and helped make this book possible, but we'd like to extend our thanks to Alicia Bunyan Sampson, Cooper S. Beckett, Dan and Dawn Williams, Amy Gahran, Carrie Jenkins, Casey Tanner, Claire Louise Travers, Ebony Hagans, Eri Kardos, Erin Tillman, Evita Sawyers, Hadassah Damien, Jaime Gama, Jessica Fern, Kathy Labriola, Leanne Yau, Libby Sinback, Dr. Liz Powell, Marie Thouin, Martha Kauppi, Michelle Hy, Rachel Krantz, Ruby Bouie Johnson, Tristan Taormino, and our hardworking team of moderators, Phi, Lore, Christina, Elizabeth, Laurel, David, Justin, Alex, Vanessa, and Nat.

And the final, biggest thanks to all our listeners and patrons who have made all of this possible. Thank you for listening, sharing, offering compassionate and kind feedback, and helping us to continue growing and improving.

EMILY'S ACKNOWLEDGMENTS

Sir Isaac Newton famously wrote, "If I have seen further, it is by standing on the shoulders of giants." For me, I am acutely aware that my achievements and success have been due to the behemoth magnanimity of those whom I am lucky enough to call my chosen family.

First, Sherry Matlack, my mom, thank you for your early edits of this book, for your endless generosity and kindness, and for always believing in and encouraging me no matter what I've wanted to do. I am supremely thankful to you for creating a safe space for me to come to you for relationship advice from an early age, and for cultivating in me a deep curiosity and desire to communicate and relate to others more healthily. Even if it was difficult at the time, I am eternally grateful for all the moments you called me on my bullshit and motivated me to get out of my own way. Your limitless influence has shaped me into the woman I am today. I love you so much, and there is no one on earth whose opinion I trust more than yours.

To my dearest and oldest friends, Tina Skrepnik and James Rappaport, you and your families (shoutout to Neb, Dragana, Christina, and Bill) have provided models of what healthy romantic relationships look like since before I knew such a thing was possible or existed. I am tremendously lucky to call the two of you my best friends. I am in awe of your brilliance, talent, and hard work. Your inspiration is boundless.

To my acting teacher and mentor Steve Eastin for educating me about life, death, instinct, self-reliance, and nonconformity.

To MC and Kim Gainey, thank you for being guiding lights in the dark tunnel that was the pandemic through the majority of writing this book. I will never tire of your stories, your humor, and your bountiful vegan food. Being your friend has truly been a gift.

To my LA vegan buddies, Jacqueline and Thaddaeus Williams,

for all the laughs, gaming, debates, and fun. You've made me a better activist and a more thoughtful person, and I have so appreciated our friendship over the years.

To Jase and Dedeker, you know me better than almost anyone, and there is truly no one else with whom I would rather write a book or spend multiple times a week producing and creating podcasts. The number of times you have lifted me back up from feelings of inadequacy and insecurity have been immeasurable, and yet you do it again and again without complaint. There aren't enough words to describe how much I care for you both or how indebted I feel to each of you. Thank you for valuing our friendships and for making this incredible creation possible.

Lastly, and most importantly, to Joshua Bennett, who has only ever been my champion throughout the entire process of writing this book, who has cheered me on time and again, held me when I cried, and celebrated all the little achievements. You have made me a better communicator, partner, and friend. You are considerate, cerebral, and introspective and challenge me to be the best version of myself. I thank you for sticking with me these past eight years through thick and thin, and for believing in the life and relationship we have created. I cherish and love you more than anything.

JASE'S ACKNOWLEDGMENTS
It turns out that writing a book is incredibly difficult and takes way more time and effort than people realize (at least more than I did!). This has been a dream of mine for years, and I have so much gratitude to everyone who made it possible.

First and foremost, Emily and Dedeker, the best possible friends and business partners I could imagine. The podcast and this book would not have been possible without the insights, input, and inspiration they bring each and every day.

A huge thank you to my many parents (bio- and step-) and my

siblings for teaching me to value both the emotional and the intellectual aspects of myself, along with a healthy balance of enthusiasm and skepticism in all things.

Erik, for asking hard questions and challenging my assumptions while still being supportive and encouraging.

The teachers and mentors who were invaluable in shaping my life. You are my heroes, and you deserve all the praise in the world.

My fellow influencers and researchers who are working to improve the diversity of research and encouraging all of us to learn from each other rather than divide ourselves further.

To Michael Bourret, a.k.a. Agent Michael, who reached out to me about writing a book after I mentioned it on a podcast episode and ended up tipping the first domino that led to this book coming into existence.

And finally, the friends and partners who have called me on my bullshit when I needed it. I probably didn't enjoy it at the time, but I think back on those experiences often with an overwhelming sense of gratitude and appreciation. Thank you for having the courage and compassion to tell me so I could learn and then share those lessons with others.

DEDEKER'S ACKNOWLEDGMENTS

They say your second baby is easier, and that's true. But damn if this wasn't a long and difficult pregnancy. First thanks has to go to my podcast coparents, Jase and Emily, for teaching me the meaning of chosen family with your patience, playfulness, and unfailing forgiveness of my faults.

Thank you to my badass author friends Jessica Graham, Rachel Krantz, and Jillian Weise. You have each inspired me, challenged me, and kept my feet on the ground. Y'all understand that writing a book is so much more than putting words on a page; you've taught me that writing a book is one part getting naked, one part bleeding out, and one part flipping the bird (by bird).

Thank you to my clients, present and past, for giving me the honor of witnessing the process.

Thank you to my agents, Uwe Stender and Brent Taylor. Thanks to Uwe for always telling it like it is, and thanks to Brent for always having the answer, in addition to lightning-fast email responses.

Thank you to the people who got me through. Thank you to Ben Day for asking thoughtful questions and listening with an open heart. Thank you to my therapists, Brian Mahan and Maiah Merino, for changing my life. Thank you to the nuns of Aloka Vihara monastery for reminding me of the way things are. Thank you to my mom, Tamra, for rising to every challenge I've thrown at you since the day we met.

References

CHAPTER 1

Conley, T.D., Piemonte, J.L. "Are There "Better" and "Worse" Ways to Be Consensually Non-Monogamous (CNM)?: CNM Types and CNM-Specific Predictors of Dyadic Adjustment." *Archives of Sex and Behavior* 50, 1273–1286 (2021). https://doi.org/10.1007/s10508-021-02027-3.

Bancroft, Lundy. *Why Does He Do That?: Inside the Minds of Angry and Controlling Men.* W. Ross MacDonald School, Resource Services Library, 2008.

Gahran, Amy. *Stepping Off the Relationship Escalator.* Booktopia, 2017.

Haupert, M. L., Amanda N. Gesselman, Amy C. Moors, Helen E. Fisher, and Justin R. Garcia. "Prevalence of Experiences with Consensual Non-monogamous Relationships: Findings from Two National Samples of Single Americans." *Journal of Sex & Marital Therapy* 43, no. 5 (2016): 424–40. https://doi.org/10.1080/0092623x.2016.1178675.

CHAPTER 2

Schaerer, Michael, Leigh P. Tost, Li Huang, Francesca Gino, and Rick Larrick. "Advice Giving: A Subtle Pathway to Power." *Personality and Social Psychology Bulletin* 44, no. 5 (2018): 746–61. https://doi.org/10.1177/0146167217746341.

Labriola, Kathy. *Love in Abundance: A Counselor's Guide to Open Relationships*. Eugene, Oregon: Greenery Press, 2010.

CHAPTER 3

Gottman, John, and Nan Silver. "The Four Horsemen of the Apocalypse: Warning Signs." Essay in *Why Marriages Succeed or Fail*. London, England: Bloomsbury Paperbacks, 2014.

Gray, John. "How to Make Peace with Cave Time in 3 Steps." MarsVenus. Accessed February 13, 2022. https://www.marsvenus.com/blog/make-peace-with-cave-time.

CHAPTER 4

Gruener, Hillary. "The One Phrase That Ends a Fight Every Single Time." https://wordfromthebird.blog/the-blog/how-to-stop-fighting-in-my-relationship/.

Ha, Priyansh. "The Magic Word Which Can Save Any Relationship Fight." https://starbiz.com/love-life/the-magic-word-which-can-save-any-relationship-fight-7172.

Laliberte, Marissa. "The Four-Letter Word That Can End Any Fight—No, Not That Word!" https://www.rd.com/article/stop-argument-one-word/.

Mackenzie, Macaela. "This Magical Phrase Will End Almost Any Argument with Your Partner." https://www.womenshealthmag.com/relationships/a19944146/phrase-to-end-fight/.

Bell, Robert A., Nancy L. Buerkel-Rothfuss, and Kevin E. Gore. "'Did You Bring the Yarmulke for the Cabbage Patch Kid?' The Idiomatic Communication of Young Lovers." *Human*

Communication Research 14, no. 1 (1987): 47–67. https://doi. org/10.1111/j.1468-2958.1987.tb00121.x.

Bombar, Meredith L., and Lawrence W. Littig. "Babytalk as a Communication of Intimate Attachment: An Initial Study in Adult Romances and Friendships." *Personal Relationships* 3, no. 2 (June 1996): 137–58. https://doi. org/10.1111/j.1475-6811.1996.tb00108.x.

Gottman, John Mordechai, and Nan Silver. *The Seven Principles for Making Marriage Work*. London, England: Seven Dials, an Imprint of Orion Publishing Group Ltd., 2018.

Morelock, Catherine Nichole. "Personal Idiom Use and Affect Regulation in Romantic Relationships." Dissertation, https:// ttu-ir.tdl.org/bitstream/handle/2346/1295/Morelock_catherine_diss.pdf, 2005.

Pearson, Judy C., Jeffrey T. Child, and Anna F. Carmon. "Rituals in Committed Romantic Relationships: The Creation and Validation of an Instrument." *Communication Studies* 61, no. 4 (2010): 464–83. https://doi.org/10.1080/10510974.2010.4923 39.

Philips, Phoebe. "The Honesty Exchange (Revisited)." Polyammering, March 27, 2017. https://polyammering.blog/2017/03/27/the-honesty-exchange-revisited/.

CHAPTER 5

Cloud, Henry, and John Sims Townsend. *Boundaries: When to Say Yes, How to Say No to Take Control of Your Life*. Grand Rapids, Michigan: Zondervan, 2017.

Google Books Ngram Viewer for "personal boundaries," Google Books. https://books.google.com/ngrams/graph?content=pers onal+boundaries.

CHAPTER 6

Collins, Lois M. "Your Husband Thinks He's Doing Equal House-work. You Probably Disagree." *Deseret News*, September 22, 2020. https://www.deseret.com/indepth/2020/9/21/21438627/american-family-survey-household-labor-division-husband-wife-children-pandemic-afs-2020-byu.

Gottman, John Mordechai. *The Science of Trust: Emotional Attunement for Couples.* New York, New York: W.W. Norton & Company, 2011.

Kauppi, Martha. "What Does It Mean to 'Hold Steady'?" Institute for Relational Intimacy, February 27, 2020. https://www.instituteforrelationalintimacy.com/blog/what-does-it-mean-to-hold-steady.

"Marriage and Couples—Research." Marriage and Couples Research. The Gottman Institute, https://www.gottman.com/about/research/couples/.

Rauer, Amy, Allen K. Sabey, Christine M. Proulx, and Brenda L. Volling. "What Are the Marital Problems of Happy Couples? A Multimethod, Two Sample Investigation." *Family Process 59*, no. 3 (2019): 1275–92. https://doi.org/10.1111/famp.12483.

Tatkin, Stan. *Wired for Love: How Understanding Your Partner's Brain Can Help You Defuse Conflicts and Spark Intimacy.* Oakland, California: New Harbinger, 2012.

Wile, Dan. "Dan's Quotes." Collaborate Couple Therapy. Accessed February 13, 2022. http://danwile.com/my-blog/my-quotes/.

CHAPTER 7

Córdova, James V., C. J. Fleming, Melinda Ippolito Morrill, Matt Hawrilenko, Julia W. Sollenberger, Amanda G. Harp, Tatiana D. Gray, et al. "The Marriage Checkup: A Randomized Controlled Trial of Annual Relationship Health Checkups." *Journal of Consulting and Clinical Psychology 82*, no. 4 (2014): 592–604. https://doi.org/10.1037/a0037097.

Irving, Alanna. "Running Agile Scrum on Our Relationship." *Medium*, July 16, 2016. https://alannairving.medium.com/running-agile-scrum-on-our-relationship-9b2085c5d747.

Morrill, Melinda Ippolito, CJ Eubanks-Fleming, Amanda G. Harp, Julia W. Sollenberger, Ellen V. Darling, and James V. Córdova. "The Marriage Checkup: Increasing Access to Marital Health Care." *Family Process* 50, no. 4 (2011): 471–85. https://doi.org/10.1111/j.1545-5300.2011.01372.x.

EXTRA TOOLS

Camras, Linda, Robert Plutchik, and Henry Kellerman. "Emotion: Theory, Research, and Experience. Vol. 1. Theories of Emotion." *The American Journal of Psychology* 94, no. 2 (1981): 370. https://doi.org/10.2307/1422757.

The Center for Nonviolent Communication, n.d. https://www.cnvc.org/.

"Clean Talk." Shadow Work, n.d. https://shadowwork.com/clean-talk/.

The Conflict Resolution (CORE) Lab, n.d. http://www.conflictresolutionlab.com/.

Driver, Janice, Amber Tabares, Alyson Shapiro, Eun Young Nahm, and John M. Gottman. "Interactional Patterns in Marital Success or Failure." *Normal Family Processes: Growing Diversity and Complexity*, 2003, 493–513. https://doi.org/10.4324/9780203428436_chapter_18.

"Everything You Need to Know about Confrontive I-Messages." Gordon Training International. Accessed February 13, 2022. https://www.gordontraining.com/leadership/everything-need-know-confrontive-messages/.

Fern, Jessica. *Polysecure: Attachment, Trauma, and Consensual Nonmonogamy.* Thorntree Press, LLC, 2020.

Gottman, John M., Janice Driver, and Amber Tabares. "Repair

during Marital Conflict in Newlyweds: How Couples Move from Attack–Defend to Collaboration." *Journal of Family Psychotherapy* 26, no. 2 (2015): 85–108. https://doi.org/10.10 80/08975353.2015.1038962.

Gottman, John Mordechai, and Joan DeClaire. *The Relationship Cure: A Five-Step Guide to Strengthening Your Marriage, Family, and Friendships*. New York, New York: Harmony, 2002.

Johnson, Sue. Dr. Sue Johnson, n.d. https://drsuejohnson.com/.

Kurdek, Lawrence A. "Predicting Change in Marital Satisfaction from Husbands' and Wives' Conflict Resolution Styles." *Journal of Marriage and the Family* 57, no. 1 (1995): 153. https://doi.org/10.2307/353824.

Penman, Maggie, and Shankar Vedantam. "Trying to Change, or Changing the Subject? How Feedback Gets Derailed." *Hidden Brain*. NPR, September 22, 2015. https://www.npr. org/2015/09/22/434597124/trying-to-change-or-changing-the-subject-how-feedback-gets-derailed.

"Consent FRIES," Planned Parenthood, August 5, 2016. https:// plannedparenthood.tumblr.com/post/148506806862/under-standing-consent-is-as-easy-as-fries-consent.

Sagiv, Lilach, Sonia Roccas, Jan Cieciuch, and Shalom H. Schwartz. "Personal Values in Human Life." *Nature Human Behaviour* 1, no. 9 (2017): 630–39. https://doi.org/10.1038/s41562-017-0185-3.

Siegel, Daniel J. *Brainstorm: The Power and Purpose of the Teenage Brain*. New York, New York: Penguin, 2015.

Walker, Pete. "The 4Fs: A Trauma Typology in Complex PTSD by Pete Walker," n.d. http://pete-walker.com/fourFs_Trauma-TypologyComplexPTSD.htm.

SPECIAL GUESTS

ALICIA BUNYAN SAMPSON is a social worker, filmmaker, and consultant based in Ontario. She is the creator and author of *Diary of a Polyamorous Black Girl*. You can find more on Instagram @polyamorousblackgirl and at polyamorousblackgirl.com.

AMY GAHRAN is the author of *Stepping Off the Relationship Escalator: Uncommon Love and Life*. Find more online at offescalator.com.

CARRIE JENKINS is a professor of philosophy at the University of British Columbia and the author of *What Love Is and What It Could Be* (Basic Books, 2017) and *Sad Love: Romance and the Search for Meaning* (Polity, 2022). Find more online at carriejenkins.net or @carriejenkins on Twitter.

CASEY TANNER is a certified sex therapist, founder of the Expansive Group, and the creator of the Instagram @queersextherapy. Find more online at theexpansivegroup.com.

CLAIRE LOUISE TRAVERS is the director of Poly Pages, an academic nonmonogamous platform. Poly Pages runs a podcast and book club dedicated to the texts that have shaped polyamorous community and culture and events hosting critical conversations about polyamory. Claire is a founding member of Polyamory Day, a national showcase of nonmonogamy in the UK and Ireland. Find more online at polypages.org, clairelouisetravers.co.uk, or polyamoryday.co.uk.

COOPER S. BECKETT is the cocreator of *Life on the Swingset: The Swinging & Polyamory Podcast* and author of several books about ethical nonmonogamy, including *A Life Less Monogamous*. Find more online at lifeontheswingset.com.

EBONY HAGANS is a pro-black polyam educator and the creator of the Instagram account @marjanilane. Find more online at marjanilane.com.

ERI KARDOS is the founder and lead love and relationships coach at Relearn Love, LLC (RelearnLove.com). She is the best-selling author of *Relationship Agreements: A Simple and Effective Guide for Strengthening Communication, Reducing Conflict, and Increasing Intimacy to Design Your Ideal Relationship*.

ERIN TILLMAN is a certified sex educator and dating empowerment coach. You can find more on Instagram @DatingAdviceGrl and online at TheDatingAdviceGirl.com/.

EVITA "LAVITALOCA" SAWYERS is the creator of "Today's Polyamory Reminder." Find more on Twitter @EvitaSawyers and on Instagram @lavitaloca34.

HADASSAH DAMIEN is a progressive financial strategist and the creator of Ride Free Fearless Money. Find more online at ridefreefearlessmoney.com.

JAIME GAMA is a psychotherapist who specializes in ethical relationships and is the creator on Instagram of @gotitasdepoliamor. Find more online at gotitasdepoliamor.com.

KATHY LABRIOLA is a nurse, counselor, and hypnotherapist in private practice in Berkeley, California, providing affordable mental health services to alternative communities including the poly, kink, sex worker, and LGBTQ communities and political activists. Kathy is author of four books, *Love in Abundance* and *The Jealousy Workbook*, published by Greenery Press, *The Polyamory Break-up Book*, published by Thorntree Press, and *Polyamorous Elders: Aging in Open Relationships*, published by Rowman and Littlefield. Find more online at kathylabriola.com.

KEVIN A. PATTERSON, MEd, is the author of *Love's Not Color Blind: Race and Representation in Polyamorous and Other Alternative Communities*. Find more on Instagram @polyrolemodels.

LEANNE YAU is the founder of Poly Philia, a page dedicated to bite-size nonmonogamy education and entertainment. Find her at @polyphiliablog on Instagram, TikTok, Facebook, and Twitter.

LIBBY SINBACK is a relationship coach and the host of the podcast *Making Polyamory Work*. Find more online at libbysinback.com.

DR. LIZ POWELL is a psychologist and the author of *Building Open Relationships*, as well as the cofounder of Unfuck Your Polyamory (with Kevin Patterson). Find more on Twitter @drlizpowell and online at drlizpowell.com.

MARIE THOUIN, PhD, is a dating and relationship coach and compersion researcher. Find more online at whatiscompersion.com.

MARTHA KAUPPI is a therapist, coach, and founding director of the Institute for Relational Intimacy. She is the author of

Polyamory: A Clinical Toolkit for Therapists (and Their Clients).
Find more online at instituteforrelationalintimacy.com.

MICHELLE HY is a polyamory advocate from Portland,
Oregon, who runs the Instagram and website Polyamorous While
Asian, which seeks to normalize nonmonogamy and promote the
voices of other POC, who are significantly underrepresented in
nonmonogamous communities. Find more online at polyam-
orouswhileasian.com.

PHOEBE PHILIPS is a relationship coach and the creator of the
blog and podcast *Polyammering.* You can find more on Twitter @
polyammering and online at polyammering.blog.

RUBY BOUIE JOHNSON, LCSW, LCDC, is a mental health
practitioner based in Texas who specializes in nonmonogamy, kink,
and infidelity. Find more online at https://www.inamorata.me.

TRISTAN TAORMINO is the author of many books, including
*Opening Up: A Guide to Creating and Sustaining Open Rela-
tionships.* She is the host of the *Sex Out Loud* podcast. Find more
on Twitter @TristanTaormino and online at tristantaormino.com.